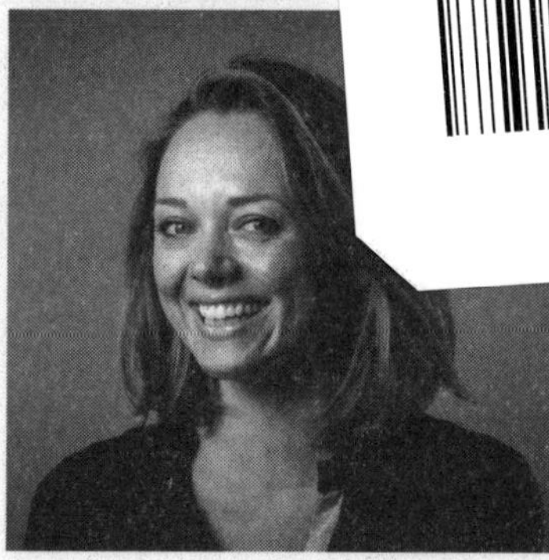

Ella Ward has worked in advertising for twenty years. This means she has a proclivity for profanity and doesn't respect punctuation. In 2018 she was hit with the cancer stick, which apart from being rather frightening also encouraged a foray into oversharing on Instagram, and then – magically – writing. Her words have been published in places like *Frankie*, *Lunch Lady*, *The Age* and *The Sydney Morning Herald*. Ella lives in Melbourne, Australia, with her husband, child, dog, cat and many (many) neuroses. She's also writing this about herself in the third person, which she acknowledges is both pretentious and a bit weird.

27 Letters to my Daughter

ELLA WARD

HarperCollinsPublishers

HarperCollins*Publishers*
Australia • Brazil • Canada • France • Germany • Holland • Hungary
India • Italy • Japan • Mexico • New Zealand • Poland • Spain • Sweden
Switzerland • United Kingdom • United States of America

First published in Australia in 2022
by HarperCollins*Publishers* Australia Pty Limited
Level 13, 201 Elizabeth Street, Sydney NSW 2000
ABN 36 009 913 517
harpercollins.com.au

A catalogue record for this book is available from the National Library of Australia

ISBN 978 14607 6042 0 (paperback)
ISBN 978 14607 1379 2 (ebook)
ISBN 978 14607 4069 9 (audiobook)

Cover design by Kristy Lund-White
Typeset in Bembo Std by Kirby Jones
Printed and bound in Australia by McPherson's Printing Group

FSC www.fsc.org MIX Paper from responsible sources FSC® C001695

For my daughter.
You are my bestest heart girl.

Contents

Letter One

Twenty-seven letters

My darling,
You're holding this book because I can no longer hold you. It feels cruel that my last act as a mother was to die. I'm so sorry. It's the one thing, more than anything, I wish I could undo.

However, as I look back on my life, there isn't much else I would change. But you'll come to see that. You'll see a lot of things, because in this book I'm giving you everything. All of it. I haven't left a bit out.

I have written twenty-seven letters for you. In them are the lessons I've learned, and earned, in my life. All 188 of them. Lessons that have come from the monsters I've vanquished, the mistakes I've made and the loves I've forgiven. The adventures I've flown. The spells I've woven. The tears I've wiped. I've sewn them all together in these pages. Every word I've written is for you: to keep you and strengthen you, and hold you, now I cannot.

I haven't written these letters alone. Did you know that our family comes with generations of words captured and chronicled? And, oh boy, are they some words! My darling daughter, you come from a family of letter-writers, nostalgists, storytellers and people who *quite like giving toasts at dinner parties*.

Or, as your great-grandmother put it to me recently, 'We are a family of people who believed they were important enough to write it all down.'

Important or not, it turns out that whatever I've been through in my life, someone else in my family has usually gone through it already. When I first began to read their words, this overlapping of experience felt like coincidence, but it soon grew into a regular occurrence. I've chosen to take great comfort in this serendipity. It means that these twenty-seven letters are not only a gift from me, but from all of us.

While everyone has a family, ours is a little more unusual than most. I hope these letters will not just hold you, in my absence, but they'll also allow you to fall in love with these unconventional ancestors. Their words of wisdom have often been a comfort to me, but their sparkles of madness have always been a cure! I believe that being brave and kind and clever is one thing – but being all those things with a twinkle in the eye is another. Which is why I cannot wait to introduce them all to you.

There's an American soldier who's fighting through Europe in 1918. There's also a woman running away from an elephant in Kenya, in the 1960s. There's a man brandishing a pistol in World War II Shanghai, and a teenager slopping through the mud on the last day of Woodstock.

These are your relatives and they all have lessons for you, to add to mine.

These letters will arm you with the knowledge, wisdom and wonder of us all. Because when push comes to shove, and death is dancing closer than you'd like, family becomes more important than anything else. We are a group of people who weren't dissuaded by little things like death. Or war. Or loss. Or elephants. I am one of them – which means, so are you.

And so, now I am done and dead and you are left with this. My all. To you, my everything.

I love you.

Mama x

Letter Two

Introductions

What sets one family apart from another? What makes your family *yours*? Is it the curve of a nose that is echoed through generations? A tinkle in a laugh that goes up and down on a scale? Or is it something less tangible: a sense, a hum in your belly, a feeling of coming home?

Family is all those things, but none of them can exist without one important element: the telling of stories. A family is only as strong as the stories that are told. And, I'm afraid to say, the stories can't just be told – they need to kept.

One afternoon, I sat down with my great-grandfather Jim's letters from World War I. Tucked away in a locked-down house in the middle of a pandemic, I found myself eyeing the innocuous-looking green ringbinder on my bookshelf. As the meme goes, 'Our grandparents had to go to war, *you* just have to sit on the couch.'

I'd been sitting on the couch. I wondered what it felt like to go to war.

Jim's letters from the Front to his sweetheart, Kay, contained extraordinary stories. But then added to them, was Jim himself. His words allowed me to live his wit, passion (raunch!), pathos and the small, curious details he was surrounded by. As I read on, Jim became more real than any sepia-dusted photograph I had seen. While we have Jim to thank for the stories themselves, it's Virginia, Jim's daughter, to whom I'm so grateful for passing them along.

Virginia, my Grama, painstakingly transcribed her father's spidery, pencil-written letters and gifted them to me way back on my twenty-fourth birthday. They languished in various houses for fifteen years. But 2020 was the year to complete my letters to you, and the year – it seemed – to read Jim's letters to everyone.

One day you're writing letters of love from the Front, the next … your great-granddaughter is reading them from beyond the dawn of the twenty-first century. There's only one reason these stories have been able to travel so easily through time: family.

This is what family is, my girl. It's a passing-on of responsibility. A collective agreement between those who sit on ever-widening branches of a family tree. An understanding that the lessons must be protected for the next generation.

Family doesn't just require a history told, it requires a history *held*, passed on, so the newest members can look back and see, with a small gasp of recognition, just what special group of people they belong to.

And this family, our family, has two very important things going for them. Yes, we've written it all down, but – crucially – we've all kept it safe for the next generation. Which is why this family can remain a home for me, and you, and for those who are still to arrive. It's how I managed to discover so many overlappings of experience. It's what has meant I can write my letters to you.

I think it might be rude to talk about people without properly introducing them. But I know it's definitely rude to publish their private letters and memoirs, their fears and dreams, near-deaths and true-loves without properly introducing them.

So. These members of your family are the ones who wrote it all down, and protected the words for the next line of the family tree.

They are my great-grandparents Jim and Kay, my Grama (Virginia) and Grampa (Buzz), my mother (Kate), and me. And, of course, we all have you. And now you have all of us.

Jim, Kay, Virginia, Buzz and Kate have all written down their stories, their letters and their lives. Over this past year I have swum around in their words and filled myself up with their histories. I am dizzy on dust and my fingers are papery from scanning.

But this isn't just a collection of old stories swept into new letters. Because anecdotes are wonderful, but they're also a dime a dozen. No, my sweet girl, I have a wonderful secret to let you in on. The tales *this* family have shared, come with a very special magic.

Bringing each of these stories together is playing five records all at the same time and realising – alarmingly – that it's all … harmonising. Is this music or is this noise? Who cares! It sounds *wonderful.*

Would you like to see how the magic works? How a family of storytellers have passed something special down the line? Come now, hold my hand, let's begin.

*

Grama. Virginia. My grandmother and probably the central reason all of these letters are here for you. The keeper of the family archives. It's fitting that she's the first voice we'll hear in these letters – other than mine, of course. The initial 'hello' comes from her own room, and it comforts me that she clearly feels as fond of her first bedroom as I am of mine. We'll check back in with Grama often enough, but there's one specific thing I want to share from this particular memory of hers, so you can begin to hear this magical harmony for yourself.

It's around 1932 and she is about five years old. We're in California. Listen:

The bathroom is all warm and steamy. Daddy's been shaving in here. I wish I'd got up in time to watch him cover his face with Ivory soapsuds and see the dent in his shoulder made by the German shrapnel. I know what shrapnel is, Daddy told me. But I don't understand a lot of things he told me about the war …

'Daddy' is James A. Quinby. That Jim in that war. My great-grandfather; your great-great. And while little Virginia was considering the divot in her father's shoulder in the 1930s, back in 1918 Jim wrote to his sweetheart Kay (Virginia's future mother), about that very scar:

… I'm glad to be moving again. They took my bandages off yesterday – entirely cured, except for a light dimple in my shoulder – won't be able to wear a low neck for a while. My letters won't be so regular – but you'll know one thing will be regular – that's – Love
… Jim.

After Jim was Jim, and Daddy, he was Grampa. Although her parents took her all around the globe, my mother, Kate, would visit her grandparents back in the USA as often as she could. In 1969 she was sixteen and dancing with her Grampa around his Palo Alto living room:

Tobacco, Ivory soap, wood polish, daphne. I try hard to stay loose-jointed and fluid … at the same time I'm concentrating on the tight-framed foxtrot. My bare foot is practically behind Grampa's brown brogues but I'm not worried. They never touch me.

Can you see the magic? You see? Many different songs but they're all blending *just right*.

This family of yours, whether by genetics or design, has interlaced the very physical manifestations of memory through its own history and lessons. I find that I have done the same. Through all of my years I can tug on a shred of smell – say, daphne on a mid-winter's afternoon – and not only will my own memories come tumbling out, but more will follow behind. Memories that aren't mine – memories I'm just holding safe to pass along. In writing these letters for you, I have come to realise time is elastic and what feels like forever ago can suddenly be very present. Life goes by so, so quickly.

Your family are people with a sense of joy, a taste for adventure, a predilection for drama and the ability to understand that 'life is a matter of contrast'. For generations we have met misfortune with a determined curiosity and even, often, genuine cheer. And all the way through, we've decided we are not only 'important enough to write it all down', but we think you are important enough for us to keep sharing.

This is why I love our family. This is why I have called upon them to help me send love to you, my daughter. This is why it's time for you to know where you have come from, and where you may be heading.

This is the first lesson for you, darling girl. Wrapped up in your very DNA is the ability to be courageous, clever and kind in the face of all kinds of fuckery.

So gather hold of those DNA strands and jump on in – the water's fine!

Lesson #1: If you have a family, you have a story.

Letter Three

You have to start somewhere

This is the letter about beginnings. About the time when generations past appeared in this world, about the time when *you* appeared in this world, and about the way some of these tales have remained, though many have disappeared.

Of the characters whose words are woven through this letter, I am the exception, for the rest of you were born in May, but I in August. A chill August day in Melbourne inside a dark Victorian hospital with red brick walls and windows that said, 'Go Away':

> *Here you are. You are here. Fleshy and silken, fingers like deep-sea anemones. Blistered lips and hair like damp feathers. So pleased to meet you. I'm your mother (mother!) … and I am at your service.*

That's my mother speaking. In August 1981 she had birthed her first child, me, and by arriving I had made the 28-year-old woman a mother. Even though I was only a few hours old, hands moving like sea creatures as if I were still floating in her belly, she was asking me those questions only a mother could ask:

Will you be happy? Will you be cautious? Will you shine? Will you love your life? I will keep you safe until you find out.

Now, forty years later, I believe it's only fair of me to answer them.

Will you be happy? – Yes. Not always, but enough.

Will you be cautious? – Yes. Always. Too much … but that caution will end up saving my life. For a time.

Will you shine? – Not immediately. But, I hope, eventually.

Will you love your life? – Yes. Yes! Most definitely. Even in the darkest days, I will love the parts of my life that are important: you, your father, the way the sun catches raindrops falling from a bridge.

So I think we can agree this means that Mum held up her end of the bargain: she kept me safe until I found all of this out. Mum asked a final question, in those grey pre-dawn hours, quiet in a room filled with new baby smells:

Do I have to share you with other people? – Of course she had to share. We all do. From the moment your baby leaves your body, you begin farewelling them. Sometimes willingly, sometimes not. It's the grief and wonder of being a mother: letting go a part of your soul.

Lesson #2: When you love something more fiercely than yourself, your greatest gift will be to let go.

Mum answered the last question herself:

Do I have to share you with other people?

Not for a long time, I hope. You need to complete your orientation first. Then you can study for your degree in Becoming a Matriarch … your B.M. The Professor Emeritus will be here in the morning, but until then, you are all mine.

The 'Professor Emeritus' was my Grama, Virginia.

Virginia, when I consider her age in 1981 (fifty-four) seems alarmingly young to be a grandmother, let alone one to be granted the title of Emeritus of the Matriarchy. But things ran younger back then, and younger even further back.

When Virginia had just turned twenty-six, she – the Professor – was only in her burgeoning years. It was 1953 and her maternal academia stretched out, unearned, before her. With one child at home, in the early hours of a May day, she welcomed her second: Kate.

> *At 3.23 am when Kate finally emerged, the doctor pulled down his mask to reveal a face grey with fatigue and covered with a day's growth of stubble. Kate had forceps scars on her head, but seemed none the worse for wear.*

I believe Grama is trying to tell us that it was a difficult labour. Aren't they all? And I wonder: if the doctor was fatigued, wasn't she? And if she was, did she say?

There's something interesting about this snippet, my girl: it's the last labour we get to hear about from the one who's experienced it. In this family story, anyway. The further back we go, the cloudier the accounts get, the murkier the records become and the more whispery the ghosts seem. This is where I will open a lesson to you that, if followed, will allow a continuing of this story.

Lesson #3: Write it down, my darling. You think you'll remember. You won't – and even if you do, the people who come after you will not.

So.

Ella was born to Kate in August, and had hair like damp feathers.

Kate was born to Virginia in May, and was marked by forceps.

Virginia was born to Katherine in May, and … and? Here comes some of that murk and clouds and whispering.

As I begin this letter to you, May has rolled around again and Virginia's ninety-fourth birthday is approaching. I emailed her, asking if her mother ever told her about the day she, Virginia, was born. Katherine (or Kay, as many called her) didn't – or if she did, Grama can't recall. She can't recall not because she's nearly ninety-four (which would be entirely understandable) but because her mother did not include that particular tale in her wider story. I assume it's because mothers did not talk of specifics then, in the 1920s. No forceps, no blistered lips. Women's physical experience rarely made it to the family lore.

This is in general. *In general* women have been quieted – their stories have often not been regarded as important enough to make it to paper. Yet in the margins of this specific family line, women have spoken louder than many of their counterparts. However, I'm afraid that there are still fewer stories from your sex than the other, even from this family of loud, wonderful women. And that may be one of the reasons why I can't share Kay's own description of childbirth with you. Even so, you are the next in a line of women who have always laughed loudly, spoken clearly and – mostly – told their story. You are allowed to continue this line. You are needed to continue this line.

Lesson #4: Whether it's blood or sweat or pain or ecstasy, tell your story. Tell it in a way that will remain.

What has seemed to survive the almost-century of time is not a visceral memory of a labour, but love instead. Grama's reply to my question was:

Mother didn't tell me about the day I was born. But [my brothers] did. Daddy left them in the car and, because it was after visiting hours, [he] climbed the fire escape of the old Palo Alto hospital to see his Beloved.

Oh Jim, climbing fire escapes up to the centre of the story he seemed to always be the hero of. Dashing Jim lived to have and tell many adventures. Which is ironic when you consider the first May of this story, Jim's birth, occurred without a paper-scratch or an ink blotch. His first appearance didn't make any story at all.

I was born in a small back-country area in Maryland, on May 28, 1895. This country was so remote and so uncivilized that they didn't think about recording the event of my birth. And that caused me, some fifty years later, a great deal of difficulty in getting a passport. Of course, there were county records of certain types of things; I imagine that a criminal trial would be recorded, but a little thing like a boy being born was like a calf being born or a foal for a horse [it was]: 'Okay, that's what happened', [and] they went on to the next thing.

I wonder if Jim took that invisible appearance, that 'Okay, that's what happened', and used it as a platform from which to scaffold his own words. He built a skyscraper of writing and poetry and sketches and anecdotes from that ephemeral base. Jim began with no words, but left thousands behind him, sung down the lines from generation to generation.

Lesson #5: An empty beginning does not mean an empty continuing.

The final May of this story, *your* May, 117 years after Jim's, is as over-reported as everything has become in the twenty-first century. When you were born there were records galore. Forms clipped onto plastic folders, and matching wrist and ankle bands checked and checked again. Everywhere you went there followed a green book that held your length and weight and circumferences and all sorts of numbers written in the curly way only nurses write: biro pen pressing too hard into the paper. And there was the digital record. An endless trail of images and videos and emails and more soft-copy missives sent all across the globe, wide and far, pinging around space via satellites, dodging meteors. You had a passport at five months old. You had your second, for your second nationality, not long after.

You are, my darling, On Record.

Back in 2012, when you were born, it was very popular to write something called 'A Birth Story'. This is an often long, always overly detailed description of how one's baby came into the world. After you were born, I wrote your birth story. It is incredibly dull.

I'm glad I did write it though, because even though it contains saccharine sentences like '… and then there were three', it also reminds me of how things rolled and what time we did what thing and … oh dear. I can't sell it, even to you, the leading lady of the story.

It really is very, very boring.

Suddenly I'm realising why our forebears' births are often relegated to a few cursory lines at the beginning of their own stories. Like Kay's, a simple statement of fact:

> *I was born three years [after my sister] on April 11, 1896, in Evanston, Illinois.*

Or, in Buzz's case, they don't even mention their own appearance in their own story until some years in.

> *… [my father] left and he didn't come back. I think there was little correspondence, if any. I can vaguely remember the first Christmas after [he] left, a card arrived with a dollar bill and that was it. The year was 1929, I was four, [my sister] was six.*

This recollection of the departure of his birth father is the first time Buzz refers to himself in his own memoir. He does not enter his own play until he is four years old, sliding in from stage left. These days we comfort ourselves by the documentation of all things. But I do wonder if little Jim – your great-great-grandfather – born on a 400-acre dairy farm with less fanfare than was given to the calves born around him – is any less or more than you are? Or Buzz, or Virginia, who have written their own stories without mention of their own births, were any more insignificant arrivals?

So here is a gift to you – the tale of how you arrived. Which means if you choose to, you'll be able to include it in your own story one day, down the line. But that will be your choice, because it is your arrival, after all.

It was May. The final May of this story. I was ten days overdue, enormous, and you were not moving. This reflected your and your father's propensity to sleep in. Even today, you do not like getting out of a warm bed in the morning, and back in 2012 you were not interested in leaving my warm womb at any time of the day.

I was induced. Labour hurt more than I could have imagined; I received drugs; and some long hours later you were on your way. Our obstetrician produced some enormous salad servers she said were forceps. I suspect they had not changed in design since they imprinted on my mother's head back in 1953. Or, to be honest, since they dragged a calf from its mother on Jim's father's dairy farm in 1895.

Back to 2012. I closed my eyes and readied myself for them, and you. Until your father checked his watch and asked if he had time to move the car. The OB looked amused, but agreed and, after shelving the salad servers, left the room for a cup of tea. Tom followed her, keen to avoid a parking ticket.

The room was empty for the first time in hours, and I closed my eyes and half-slept. I was conscious of my breathing while you rearranged yourself inside my body, warm and floating, ready to join us all in the cold, dry wonderful world. I wish I'd acknowledged the last moments of our fleshy, organic intimacy a little more. Instead, I was exhausted and my body hurt. This ended up being a sound representation of my first six months of motherhood. I wish I'd appreciated that foggy newborn time more. Instead, for endless weeks, I was exhausted and my body hurt.

But on this May morning I didn't know about those months to come, I didn't even know about the minutes to come. I decided to work on the seconds. There was a small window over my right shoulder and I peered out at a blushing mauve sunrise. I was reminded of Roald Dahl and the 'pink and purple flowers of the tinkle-tinkle tree'. Music played. We'd had a whole playlist, but like the rest of labour, we couldn't time everything perfectly and you were born to Paul Kelly singing about cities in Texas.

The room filled with people again and I roused myself, turning from the tinkle-tinkle sunrise to concentrate on meeting my child.

You were born. Tom declared you a boy because he mistook the umbilical cord for a penis. The doctor gently corrected him while handing him scissors to snip said ~~penis~~ cord. Paul Kelly finished. I pulled you onto my chest.

Your head was squished and puffy, like you'd 'been through the wars' – which is not an inaccurate description of my vagina. You had forceps marks, too, curved red lines across your temples which only much later I winced at, thinking of the force with which they must have been applied. Your eyes were enormous, glossy and black. You had sea anemone fingers and hair like wet feathers. I was terrified. I was relieved. I was so tired.

And then there were three.

Letter Four

Tuck yourself in

My childhood bedroom was the first place that I created of my own; the first place where I was creative on my own. I think it's a place I've gone about trying to reconstruct ever since.

Some things remained constant through the two decades I called that room mine. The grass matting floor and the noodled lumps it left on my skin when I was kneeling on it: earlier, playing with my Barbie dolls; later, thrusting grimly through exercises when I thought my body needed toning and angles. I must have looked like a Tweeny Communist PE teacher.

Lesson #6: Don't do squats in your bedroom when you're fifteen. You don't need to. I promise.

I was four and I started with a single bed. It had 'I ❤ AUSTRALIA' printed on the mattress, and the blanket on the end of it matched that of the doll's in the bassinet beside me. My mother was clever like that. Over the bed hung a waxed canvas blind with a timber ring that needed to be pulled *just so.* Over the grass matting there was a blue and yellow Persian rug with a patch eventually worn threadbare … probably from all of those squats. A bookshelf hung at the top of my bed, creating a hidden space over my head for pictures and poetry. Eventually there was a white desk. A spinny chair. A narrow wardrobe with a delicately shuttered door.

It was small and old and very cosy.

All through my childhood, my Grama also slept in a small, old and cosy bedroom. She had a single bed under a frosted white lampshade in a shingled house near the sea. When we visited for the weekend ('a single mother's weekend spa', Mum called it) I would pull on my scratchy woollen dressing gown in the hush of the early morning and pad downstairs to join her.

She once wrote, of those mornings:

> *One of the best times of the day. Lying on my pillows, a tea tray on the bedside table and a good book in my hands. The froth of jasmine round the window motionless on this still morning. The house quiet until, like mouse scrabblings, the sound of a grandchild at the door.*
>
> *One of the best times of life. A warm, small child snuggling into bed beside me, her favourite book pushed under my nose. 'Read!' she orders, then 'please, Grama' an afterthought.*

I'm pleased to hear that I knew my manners back in 1987. We would have been reading *My Naughty Little Sister* and drinking 'Children's Cuppa Tea', which was made deliberately syrupy with an entire tablespoon of sugar, and served in a delicate china cup and saucer with tiny violets painted on the sides.

This act of sacrament wound its way deeply into my sense of what a Grandmother and her Grandchild do. We were connecting over ceremony and routine and a quiet understanding, all tucked in neatly beneath a hand-embroidered patchwork blanket. Those mornings taught me how the Expected is so very important, when you are a child.

Lesson #7: A healthy childhood comes from a place of knowing where you are, and what comes next. Don't be afraid to give that when the time comes.

Grama herself had quiet routines wound into her own childhood, beginning in her own bedroom. Back in the 1930s, she woke each morning under the peeling green kalsomine paint.

> *It's cold in the room but warm under the covers. My ruffly curtains look like ballet dancers when they move. I can hear a bird singing in the lilac, I think it's a towhee. Now I hear Mother talking and Daddy walking around. He's coming in to close my window and turn the heater on.*

She heard the same three sentences every morning:

> *'Up an' at 'em!'*
>
> *He always says that and now he's gone into the boys' room and called, 'Hit the deck!'*
>
> *The heater smells of burning dust because we haven't used it for a while ... The boys are coming down the hall toward Mother and Daddy's room.*
>
> *'What's for fruit, Mom?'*
>
> *They have to help with breakfast, fix the juice or melon and set it on the table. All I have to do is dress myself. I'd better hurry. They're always telling me to hurry. Oh! The linoleum floor is cold. Mother says it isn't linoleum, it's a linoleum rug. It looks like a big pink and green rug and has little bumps all over it. When I push clay on it then lift it up it makes a pattern on the clay ...*

Patterns in clay, bumps on knees, if we're starting here who knows where we might end up. My head is fuzzy and we've barely begun. This is what you should get used to, though. This is your family. This is the alchemy. This is time travel.

And so we fly, back to the late twentieth century. I had two doors in my bedroom, one to enter and leave from – and another, from which you could access the last room in the house – the office.

Mum, a freelancing single mother who didn't (couldn't?) say no to a job, worked into the late hours in that little room. She was crafting, ideating and illustrating advertising concepts. I'd often fall asleep to the sound of her Pantone Letraset markers squeaking across her drawing pad, the faint smell of acetone mixing in with the Nescafé. It was 1990 and I was understanding that work was Important.

My bedroom sat above the kitchen, and long dinner parties played beneath me. Mum was unfurling again after the trauma of divorce, and new (and old) friends huddled around her while my younger brother and I slept upstairs. One night, I woke to Mum and her mate softly playing guitar at the end of my bed. He had been the singer and drummer in Aussie band Daddy Cool. One day you'd dance to his bandmate playing bass at our local market. There's that time-twisting alchemy again.

The room received offerings like an altar. If Mum was out, she'd often bring home items from her journeys and leave them at the foot of my bed as I slept. Waking in the morning I'd be greeted with gifts from her other life as an artist and woman and someone who wore hairspray to parties. Helium ballooned bunches taken from an awards-night table. Silver-foiled fancy chocolates that I ate early in the morning before anyone else woke up. They were postcards from the places that Grown-Ups Went To.

Early on, the room was filled with dolls and stuffed toy animals. Of course, like every child, I knew each one's name and personality. I started a habit of doling out individual goodnight kisses, my lips pressing on furry noses and plastic foreheads. Like many habits, this soon developed into a ritual that was difficult to leave behind.

Over a period of years my mother and her parents also slept with a series of animals, across east and west Africa. Often in tents. Once, up a tree. Buzz described their treehouse bedroom:

> *Each one of the rooms had a window looking out on to this pond so that even after you'd stayed up until, say, eleven or twelve o'clock at night watching from the verandahs, you could get into bed and fix your pillows so that you could continue watching the animals well into the dawn if you wished. And they came. Elephants, rhino, water buffalo, all sorts of antelope … unbelievable.*

Grama wrote of the same night:

> *We were awed by the repeated battering given and received by two mean old rhinos. First a snort, a sideways toss of the head then a thundering gallop climaxed by an earth-shaking crash of horn on horn. Even when we finally tore ourselves away from the observation platform and crawled into our beds, we couldn't resist resting our chins on the window sill and watching the milling herds below. We were lulled to sleep by those two old rhinos still hammering at each other.*

I too would rest my chin on my windowsill some evenings, but rather than rhinos, it was growling possums shaking the ivy so hard that dust would powder the ground below.

As I edged towards teenagedom, the burgeoning compulsiveness of my toy-kissing bled into prayer, something I kept up until you were born. Actual, literal prayer. To be clear: I am in no way religious, just *very* dramatic. So I used to kneel on that grass matting and resolutely chant through the shopping list of people I needed to check in on, lest they fall off the perch while I slumbered. It was an emotional tic that became a solemnised comfort blanket. Sometimes I'd crawl into bed, forgetting to do my dues. Sighing, I'd always get back out. I didn't want someone to die overnight – or at least, I didn't want to be responsible for it.

I'm not sure where the compulsions came from. Some textbook therapy would point to something or other about 'control'. I've always tried to ward off the spirits that hovered in my periphery. Around the time you were born, I stopped the prayers, but soon another quirk became a compulsion and I found myself wishing upon the first star I saw at night. Each time, I'd wish for health and happiness, for you and me and everyone. Slightly more magical, but no less constrictive.

The day I was diagnosed with cancer, I stopped wishing on stars. Cancer cured my compulsions. There's no room for superstition when something bad happens to you. It's wonderfully freeing. Consider this when you next 'touch wood', or do something else because you feel you have to.

Because your father and I both have these tendencies, receive this letter as a sign that you can take your hands off life's remote every now and again. It's okay. I say so.

Lesson #8: It can be wonderfully freeing to realise you are not in control.

Right. Where were we? Ah, my bedroom.

Despite the above, I don't want you to think this room was a cage of obsessive compulsions. It was a very safe, special place. The spinny chair, the overflowing pinboard and the sash window that opened out into the oleander trees.

I can't say this very often now, but back then, in that room, I knew where everything was. Every corner became a nook for my secrets. Long letters with spidery writing bulged out of shoeboxes under my bed. Diaries and scrapbooks, still among my most treasured items (you better not have thrown them away – I WILL HAUNT YOU), received reverential treatment on the Best Shelf. It was like living inside a physical manifestation of my own mind, a ship's cabin secured against gales and storms. It was safe, and known, and watertight.

*

Jim wrote of many bedrooms. I met my great-grandfather once when I was very little, too young to remember much more than the smell of his pipe. But luckily for me – for you, for all of us – he left many words behind. You may have guessed he was a military man by that way he roused his children twenty years later … 'Up an' at 'em!' Did you know he went to war? The first world war. It was 1918, he was twenty-three and he sailed off in a ship as an officer. He wrote extraordinary letters back to his love and I've read every syllable over and over.

In all his letters home, what strikes me most is how many times Jim describes where he slept. Every time he beds down somewhere new he shares the details of his chamber with his love Kay: a ship's cabin, gilt and upholstered like a lady's boudoir. The recess of a stone wall in a French chateau, behind thick silk curtains. The bottom bunk of a captured German dugout. Under a machine gun carriage on a moving train. A dripping tent. A hospital room. A safe post-armistice attic:

> *There are many creature comforts even in the houses of the villages. Their beds are works of art. Mine is built into a recess of the wall and shaded by draped curtains. It is about as high as an American table and if one ever fell out of it on the stone floor he'd sure make a dent on it. The Madam puts a huge feather pillow, covered with lace and silk, on the bed each morning despite the fact that I take it off each night. There are a lot of queer customs I will tell you about when I come back.*

With all these descriptions, I like to think it's because Jim knew the importance of a bedroom. How it is the place to tuck yourself into yourself, surrender to the night, let your mind finally hear itself think. He found – in the midst of unimaginable fear, pain and horror – genuine delight in a place to sleep.

Lesson #9: Please always try to carve out a place to be safe.

I very much hope that for you this is always a physical space, but what Jim teaches us is, as long as you start out with a safe room, and you have dreams, you will always have somewhere to go back to.

> *Lord, Lady, I'd give my last tin of bully beef to see you. That's the highest compliment I can pay you for I've been carrying that tin of BB for some time. You know, my heaven used to be composed of limousines, soft music and ladies wearing pearl earrings and wings. It is now my firm conviction that Heaven is a dry place where one can sleep.*

May you always have dreams composed of limousines, soft music and ladies wearing pearl earrings and wings. Or technicoloured sun loungers, gardenia-scented nights and friends wearing twinkles and song. Whatever carves out your special place.

I learned how to properly dream in my first bedroom. I found hot nights were the best times for fantastical wonderings, after the brick walls had heated up and weren't going to cool down for days. Outside was dark but the city was alive. I'd lie awake by the open window and listen to the sounds through the flywire. Hot nights always sound different, don't they? Even now I have an aversion to sleeping through summer swelters with the windows closed and the chemical iciness of the air-conditioning slicing through the room. Up until I left home, every summer I'd fall asleep to tram squeals, cicadas and, for some years, a rehearsing saxophone.

Lesson #10: A saxophone is one of the few instruments that sound better in rehearsal than in performance.

I heard this particular instrument's notes for years. I used to go searching – the closest I came to locating the source was a window above the doctor's surgery across the park. Sometimes I dreamed that the saxophonist and I would fall madly in love. I dreamed about falling madly in love with lots of imaginary men, in that room. I would write paragraphs describing my meeting – the gentlemen would inevitably have curly hair, big blue eyes and (after one summer watching too many European films) an accent. Even then I was a premature nostalgist. Alongside the subtitles, I was watching too much Billy Wilder and reading too much John Cheever. I was yearning for what I imagined hot city nights contained for grown-up ladies about town: sitting on stoops, smoking cigarettes, wearing hats unironically and listening to jazz.

Do that for me, will you? On a hot night, open your windows as wide as a yawn and listen to the sounds roll in. Jazz, hats, stoops, etc. But maybe hold off on the ciggies.

I kept growing up. The room stayed with me. The single bed became a double – it was rescued from my grandparents' flat and sunk like a hammock in the middle. I didn't care. I was thrilled – a double bed represented another page-turn towards the chapters of my impending adulthood. The dolls, the teddies, the bassinet – they disappeared. The pinboard groaned with Annie Leibovitz photographs and restaurant matchbooks. I started burning incense and listening to music without lyrics.

Late, very late, after stomping through bars and nightclubs in plastic shoes I would sit at my desk and write poetry. Actual poetry! In pencil, on homemade paper. It felt Important. Though in my twenties, looking back, it felt Excruciating. Now, older again, it is back to Important. Most of the poetry still sits across various notebooks, but some I tore free and slid between the pages of the vintage children's books that sat on the shelf. Even today, cracking one open can release a fluttering wing of paper and verse.

Lesson #11: Make sure you keep the poetry you write as a teenager.

(Because you will write it, I promise you will.) It may be the best poetry you ever write. Maybe because it'll be the only poetry you ever write, but still …

That room held my first true heartbreak. It worked its way through me like a virus as I lay tucked like a comma in that dipping mattress. I was twenty-one, bruised with the shock of infidelity. But less than a year later those same walls shimmered with electricity as I experienced my first true love affair. A mirror hung on the wall – bevelled blue edging with faded glass. One early January evening I stood at that mirror and applied sticky pink lip balm before heading off to meet a boy. I stared at my face long enough that I began to see what others did. It was 2003 and I was realising I could control what plot twist my life next took. The room sighed after me as I left. Because that night was the beginning of a longer, permanent departure.

I was gifted a wall of this bedroom once, sent from 16,000 kilometres away. When I was living in London, Mum had a photographer mate take a large-format photo of it, printed it up on heavy vinyl and sent it over the seas. I was dumbfounded, the enormous postal tube appeared in my dark basement flat and as I unrolled it, I unrolled my bedroom. My real bedroom. I pinned it up and, like a portal to home, it took me to where I had come from, and what I missed.

I've returned twice to that room, as a guest rather than an owner. The first was after I left your father behind in England. Homesickness had become too much to bear. In a gesture that was too abrupt and too extreme to come from anyone other than an overconfident twenty-six-year-old (sorry, dear Tom) – I left. Back to the grass matting, the bevelled mirror, the pinboard in real-life 3D. It was March so the oleander still bloomed pink, the tram squealed, the bed dipped. It wasn't my room anymore.

The final iteration of my bedroom is as your bedroom. You've slept in this room from a baby. You know it. Not the way I've described it, but the shadows are there. The grass-matting has been replaced by practical carpet. The dresser moved and a cot replaced it. But you napped, pink-cheeked and farting under that same bevelled-edged mirror. And for all of those early-year snoozes, my mum, your Gaga, sat in that same office. No more Pantone felt-tips; instead her computer stylus sweeping across the pad. I'm not sure what time-travelling headtwist it must be for her to see her daughter and her granddaughter sleep in that room. Those oleander flowers. That sash window.

*

There is something very powerful about a childhood bedroom. Those four walls took me from two to twenty-two. A ship's cabin, keeping me safe as we crested and fell.

Know this: I, and all those who came before me, still remember the paint and the curtains and the feeling of the floor beneath our toes. It is indelible. This is what a childhood bedroom is, and becomes – before your world stretches out over new horizons. Make sure you remember yours and what it gave you.

In 1918, when Jim was sailing from the US to Europe, he was in the beginning-days of his correspondence and of his war. Battle had not yet commenced and so he had time to 'muse on things which catch my fancy'. He wrote from the warship he travelled on:

> *Here [this ship] is, a great, docile many colored fabric of steel and wood, plowing along with a load of husky farmer boys from*

the Pacific Coast. For the past two years she's dodged torpedoes in three oceans and carried troops to France, England and Mesopotamia. This cabin is a gilt and upholstered affair, with white panels where, no doubt, tourists and pleasure parties, India bound, have enjoyed themselves in days gone by. Over yonder, by those mauve curtained windows where Capt. Downing gracefully drapes his booted and gun-circled bulk, some fair damsel passed the time while the fans whirled above her and servants glided noiselessly in and out – Oof! I grow poetic. I apologise.

Lesson #12: Never apologise for growing poetic.

Letter Five

Your lineage is salty

Your lineage is salty. It burbled up, glowing with phosphorescence off the bow of a warship. It has been sprinkled by storm-fuelled waves sneaking through keyholes. It is decorated with salt crystal tattoos on sunburned legs.

All of this family have salt in their veins, but the only true seafarer in this crew was Jim – who at seventeen, quite literally, ran away to sea:

> *During summer vacation of my second year in high school – 1912, when I was 17 – I decided that conventional education was not for me [and] I would run away to sea … I wandered along the Baltimore waterfront and finally got a job as galley boy on the steamer Juniata, operated by [the] 'Merchants and Miners Transportation Company'. I dropped my parents a card, telling them what ship I was on, and stating that I would come home after I had achieved my ambition to see the world.*

Jim did come home, but it seems a little sooner than he expected. Being the youngest member of the crew, Jim learned about seafaring 'the hard way'. Which by his account included being promoted to deckhand (good) and engaging in a bar brawl with another ship's crew in Boston Harbor (not so good):

This ruckus was more serious. All hands were throwing beer mugs. The police came, and I was afraid they'd toss me in the pokey, so I climbed out a window, and ran off into the sand dunes … Later, when I came back, everything was dark, and the last trolley car had left for Boston. I hung around until daybreak, and got back to the waterfront on the first car.

My ship had sailed.

Lesson #13: Do not run away to sea at seventeen.

Jim saw that steamer again six years later, when he was aboard a different ship and achieving that ambition to see the world – although maybe not in the way he'd hoped or planned.

This is our fifth day out and we haven't sighted a sail. Must be off the beaten track. Coming out of harbor we passed the 'Juniata' M & M. Co. boat on which I [last] sailed in 1913. It gave me a queer turn to see her. Lots of things around the East Coast give me a queer turn – kinda pull at my memory.

It was July 1918, America was at war, and he was headed out to fight in Europe.

Last night I was on duty part of the time as Officer of the Guard on deck … This watch on the bridge is an eerie job. The convoy sails at night without lights and it's a matter of plunging ahead in the blackness and keeping your eyes open. It's there on the bridge, with the darkness so heavy that you can't see the bow of the ship and the waves breaking into phosphorescence seventy feet below, that you realise what a job the navigators have.

Jim wrote this to Kay as he sat at a cork-topped table in the ship's smoking room. As he said, 'It's hard to believe we're in any danger', but then, he was also keenly aware that previous ships on the same trip over had been torpedoed by the enemy. Which is why the convoy sailed at night without lights and the 'Sergeant of the Guard persist[ed] in seeing imaginary craft on our starboard quarter every half hour, and call[ed] me to look'.

> *This walking up and down the length of a darkened ship is a funny thing ... The deck, covered with sleeping men and bulky in the shadows with ventilators and machinery, stretches away forward. The great stacks tower above and roll and pitch against a cloudy sky just beginning to be light in patches. The sea, torn and choppy in the grey light, spreads around.*

It was not the last time Jim was at sea, but it was certainly the most dangerous.

When Kay had met Jim in 'the Fall of 1916 at a campus dance', she was living with her family in Long Beach, California. Kay tells us about this place, where she slept under shingles by the sea:

> *My father built a two-storied brown shingled house on Cedar Avenue, Long Beach. Long Beach in 1905 was a little town with a beautiful beach where we enjoyed playing in the sand and bathing in the ocean.*

The sea can be beautiful and bathed-in, or it can be deep and dark. Another war and another young man: this time Jim's son-in-law Buzz, before he had a chance to fall in love with Virginia. In the next world war, the most dangerous ship for Buzz was the one he did not sail upon:

> *I got my commission [as an officer]. I was still nineteen. My orders came through [and] I was to report to [the United States Pacific*

Fleet] in Hawaii. There were six of us with the same orders ... [and] when we checked in at the Admin Office I noticed the clerk put my file in a different drawer than the other five guys.

In about five days they were shipped out. I wasn't in a hurry and finally [my adopted mother] brought [my then fiancée] up to San Francisco for a visit, and chaperoned us. After thirty days I got bored and went back to the administration office.

I reported in every morning and every morning I said, 'Well, when am I going?'

Finally the clerk said, 'Good God. I put your file over here and forgot about you.'

So they pulled my file out and I went to Hawaii.

The other five guys were dead. They all got there just in time to get assigned to destroyers, which is what they wanted, and they got into the big Kamikaze action.

Lesson #14: Sometimes it can pay to be forgotten.

While the rest of us are not officers guarding the deck, or waiting for our drawer to be opened, we are a family who have long embraced how powerfully the sea can impact our souls. Luckily, both Jim's and Buzz's treacherous beginnings did not colour how they – or the rest of this family – felt about the salty deep.

I started my journey with the ocean in a little hamlet called Point Lonsdale, on Victoria's Bellarine Peninsula. Buzz and Grama had bought a shack there in 1970. As Buzz said:

One of the reasons we picked this particular spot is because we could walk. It's 1100 feet to the surf and 1100 feet to the shops. I didn't like the idea of having to get into your car to go to the beach. To me that spoilt it. I used to walk to the surf beach to go body surfing.

There is a photograph of Buzz bodysurfing. He looks like a sleek walrus emerging from the foam, arms stretched behind him, water streaming from his form. He was famous for the lengths the waves took him (or he them). When I was little and Buzz seemed even bigger than he actually was, I wondered why he was never afraid of the sea. Never afraid, even when it was torn and choppy, and even when the waves seemed big enough to swamp his solid frame.

But I needn't have worried. When he was a teenager in California, Buzz rode waves bigger than the ones in Bass Strait, 1100 feet from his beach shack door.

> *We had a tidal wave on the main beach at Laguna. I was out body surfing and the beach was very crowded. I think it was a weekend. I was looking towards the beach and I saw everybody get up and run. I looked around and this huge wave was coming. It was dead calm so it was something that happened out at sea. I swam towards it but it didn't break. I went right up to the top of it. I looked back and saw people still running from the beach and the wave went right across the beach and into the main street, taking towels and umbrellas with it.*

While Buzz was born in Arkansas, at seven years old he moved to California to live with his aunt and uncle, who became his adopted parents. They were much wealthier than his birth mother back in the south, and soon Buzz and his sister were living in a lovely shingled home in Busch Gardens, Pasadena. There was a beach house, too – that hung over that ocean at Laguna Beach and where the water came through the keyhole of his bedroom door when there were storms.

I hope Buzz felt as safe in that house then as we did, my younger brother and I, when ocean storms buffeted our bedroom in Point Lonsdale. The room that we slept in as children, which Buzz and Grama always called the Nursery, was really just a box perched atop the beach house, which by the time we were born had a roof covered in more shingles. These Buzz had hammered in by hand. The house was a unique labour of love that grew to be much more than the original fibro shack they had bought years before I was born. They called it Shenzi.

> *People ask, 'What have you been doing in your retirement?' I like to work with my hands. I've been working on this house since 1970. Plans were that when I retired I would add a big 700-square-foot extension myself. And I did. The house was a wreck so there was a lot of general maintenance to do all the time. I've replaced twenty-seven windows and sixteen doors. [When we first arrived] the house was a mess. Now it is quite liveable.*

On nights when winter storms rolled into Port Phillip Bay, my brother and I would lie in our narrow beds and listen to the waves crash on the beach with such violence that I feared we'd be carried away. Sometimes the lighthouse's foghorn would add its tune, a mournful lowing over the tea-trees. Mornings after, the sun would rise through wet windows. We would set off on seaweedy walks, picking our way along the surf beach through dark-green shreds of kelp with roots thicker than my thigh. As Grama always said, the only time it is acceptable to sniff is during a beach walk on a cold morning. Anything powerful enough to tear those enormous rubber trees from the depths made me uneasy. I would sniff all the way from the surf club to the lighthouse, inhaling that overripe ocean smell.

You know that walk well, and I have repeated Virginia's lesson to you often. You sniff all the way to the lighthouse, too.

*

Once winter has blown into the other hemisphere, the surf beach – or the Back Beach, as we call it – changes. In the summertime, the beast of the beach calms. The foghorn is silent and the kelp remains more or less where it belongs: anchored deep below. Vast flat rocks stretch out into the break and at low tide hold deep pools of fishy magic.

My brother and I would spend *days* down there as kids, Mum keeping an eye from the sand while we fossicked and discovered and bickered and sang. There was one pool that held its own underwater tunnel. Mum was forty-two when we made her get in. I didn't realise until recently that she was worried she wouldn't get out:

This should be easy. Exhale first – important – now inhale deeply. Now, crouch and push off along the floor of the rock pool toward the curtain of seaweed. Swim through it into the tunnel, kicking like hell. It's waaay darker than I expected. 'What if I get stuck? What if I drown here in front of my horrified children?' I kick harder. The tunnel narrows and kelp fingers tickle my sides, my legs, and grab my ankles. Oh dear Jesus.

Another curtain of seaweed parts and I'm bathed in sunlight. I break through the surface and exhale.

'Yay! She DID it!'

'Woah Mum! Kick ASS!'

Those long hot Lonsdale beach days smelt of suncream and tasted of a meat pie crunched with sand. They were some of the first days our newly diminished family of three understood that we would be okay. As Jim would say, it was a matter of 'plunging ahead in the blackness and keeping your eyes open'. Mum kicked harder. We cheered her on. And together we emerged, bathed in sunlight, beginning to heal.

Where you and I are concerned, my girl, the torn-grey Atlantic Ocean and the kelpy-deep of Port Phillip Bay are just the beginnings of a sea-sewn tapestry made for healing. We've added our own thread to the briny fabric – a crystallised turquoise of tropical waters.

I believe there's something particular about the equatorial air that makes you and me happy, my girl. I recall the first time you experienced the humidity of the tropics, and your father as well. Tom grew up with the mild heat of England and the dry heat of Spain. Englishmen don't tend to get to the South Pacific like we Aussies do.

So you were only three when you first stepped through the plane's hatch onto the airstair. You pinched your little fingers through the humid afternoon air and said, 'Mama! The air is wet. The air is heavy!'

When my mother, Kate, was five, she stepped out into Hawaii and had her own first wonderment at the magic that is the humid face-slap of an equatorial plane landing:

> *The air is juicy. It smells of frangipani flowers and engine fuel. We climb out of the plane and step down the hot stairs onto the shimmering tarmac ... Vines cover everything, even the buildings. The birds make so much noise we can't hear each other. More frangipani, more gardens and more smiling people ... We drink special drinks and eat special food. More dancing, more singing, more smiling. Everyone in my family is smiling.*

Years later and our family have found a special place, an island speck in the Coral Sea, where we too smile all the time.

The first time I visited this island was in the 1980s, when my family was still 'Mum, Dad, two kids': a nuclear foursome. We were as invincible and as doomed as an atomic reactor. I don't remember much of that trip except the smell of the frangipani flowers, the breakfast buffet, and the lack of worry about the future.

Even so, I was shy to go back; to introduce you and Tom to something that mightn't live up to the blurred memories I'd kept.

But when I returned thirty years later, you both in tow, the little Fijian island was just the same. The same air, the same frangipani, the same smiles.

We even took a photo, you and I, standing in the very spot that my dad and I had stood decades earlier. I exclaimed over this overlapping to the staff at the time but they didn't seem as surprised as I expected. After all, they had been there fifty years. They'd seen three, four … *five*! … generations of many families do the same thing. I was time travelling in a place that was filled with time travellers. And now it was our turn to make the island our own, and sew the sea into our memories.

We have been back a number of times, before the coronavirus pandemic closed the world to us. The last time we visited I was only months past completing cancer treatment. All year, through pain and chemicals and fire, I had been meditating over our moment of arrival. Of the evening gloam giving way to inky sky, when the small boat would heave onto the sand of that little beach, and we'd pull off our shoes to wade the last few metres ashore. With the salt crystals already drying tight on our knees, the waves would gently buffet the boat behind us.

That first moment, when our travel-tired feet hit the warm water, is the closest I think I'll ever come to baptism.

The English say everything is better after a hot cup of tea. I say, few problems aren't lessened by dipping bits of yourself into the ocean. You and I have bobbed, floated and skimmed in the greens, blues, sparkles and foams of three different oceans. Your people have sailed over thousands of kilometres of sea. We have been dumped by waves and we have swept along shores. There is salt in our veins.

Remember my darling, no matter where or when you are, if you go to the water's edge and smell the salt, I will be there too.

Lesson #15: When in doubt, go to the sea.

Letter Six

Say 'I do', or say 'I don't'

Between them, my parents have been married eight times.

How's that for a one-liner? I'm not proud to say that I've rolled it out at a dinner party or two. But you know, like I do, it's not a breezy quip. It's eight Hopes and Promises and Six Sadnesses and Endings. It's heartbreak. It's betrayal. It's me, sitting in the McDonald's car park with my dad, wondering how to make him feel less awkward about leaving my mother. I was eight years old.

My grandparents (your great-grandparents), both sets, were married until the end. Married early, married endlessly, until one of them was no longer. The curious thing about marriages 'back then' is how simple we all think they were. When Grama spoke of marrying Buzz (who as well as 'Buzz', shared the same name as her father – Jim), she acknowledges this:

> *We'd been going out only five or six weeks that fateful day of the picnic in the Stanford foothills. Following our hike we'd stopped at Hank's, a bar on Bayshore Highway, where we'd had a couple of martinis and met a well-dressed couple of friends who were on their way to the city.*
>
> *'If you can be back here in half an hour we'll go up together.'*

> *Jim drove me home, proposed, I accepted, he went somewhere to change, I rushed inside for my shower and momentous conversation with Mother before leaving for the city.*

I'd like to know what Kay said when her daughter burst in, a martini down, and en route to the shower told her, 'Jim proposed!'

> *Present emotions are difficult enough to analyse but to slip back fifty years and try to recreate my feelings then toward Jim is all but impossible. Why did I accept his proposal of marriage? Why did he want to marry me? There was the physical attraction – but to be honest, I found most men attractive.*
>
> *I suppose we were both relying heavily on instinct.*

Ha! Grama! 'To be honest, I found most men attractive.' She's right though. It could be that with decades of both success and hindsight, a marriage appears an easy simplicity. One that was merely borne from the result of being young and (apologies Grama) just a bit … randy.

But the other point she makes rings more closely to truth: 'relying heavily on instinct'. There's a lot to be said for the deep-down hum in your gut that tells you if you're making the right decision. I am not sure at what point I decided I was going to marry your father. It was after he moved to Australia, but well before he proposed. Those two landmark moments bookended what was, if I really consider it, also just instinct.

If I think back to my first real love affair at twenty-two, the one before your father … well. Who am I to judge Buzz and Virginia? If the world was as wild in 2003 as it must have felt in the heady flush of those just-postwar years, then I expect marriage would have come as easily to me as it did to my grandparents. Particularly after a hike and a martini.

Buzz's account of the same proposal is similar, if a little more perfunctory:

... Virginia was sitting there on a day bed looking a million dollars. I knew her only vaguely at Pomona [College]. She looked great – she had a grey skirt on with pockets and a long sleeved red blouse. She had her own car and was a juvenile probation officer – she had majored in sociology. Her headquarters were in San Jose. I hit it off with 'Quig' as we called her. We liked each other from the start. We were only going out for six weeks when I gave her a double martini, proposed and she said yes.

Grama's elaboration:

For both of us the biological clock had struck. This isn't as unromantic as it sounds; both of us were ready for the challenges, delights and security of marriage.

Virginia and Buzz were full of martini and excitement about getting married, something their respective parents will have needed to catch up on. We don't know what Virginia's parents thought, but she tells us what process her future in-laws had to move through:

[Buzz] wasn't perfect when it came to filling in his own parents with regard to his plans. When we became engaged I suggested he write his parents in New York, telling them the news before it was in the paper. He wrote a brief note, omitting to tell them my name or anything about me. His poor mother groaned to his father: 'He's had a biological urge in a hamburger joint and has to marry her.'

One evening at a dinner party [his mother] was seated next to a New York attorney and poured out her anxieties to him.

'Who knows what the boy's got himself tangled up with.'

'What did you say the girl's name was?'

'Virginia Quinby.'

'Is her father an attorney in San Francisco?'

'Yes, I think so.'

'Well, if Jim Quinby is allowing your son to marry his daughter, you can count yourself lucky.'

And that's why I know that it wasn't just youth, beauty, grey skirts and a healthy libido. These children, barely adults, were growing up around war and a Depression, between famine and fear. They were falling in love and lust in an era when safety and security meant more than it had for a long time. To understand this swiftly pushes the concept of marriage and what it used to stand for into sharp relief. They were not babies; they were young people who had already witnessed a lifetime of loss. It's a reminder that makes me feel better about not settling down with my One True Love. Especially because that One True Love did not end up being my One True Love. But instead One (of my) True Loves.

Lesson #16: Marriage isn't the scripted ending (or beginning) people will lead you to believe.

Even Buzz and Virginia's marriage, bedded in family lore as something close to Camelot, is a union neither you nor I might want in these so-called 'modern' times:

From the beginning Jim led, I followed. Occasionally I felt minimised but most of the time I was willing for Jim to make the decisions, worry over finances, and laugh at my limitations. We were in love until the day he died.

You and I, my love, might wince at the politically incorrect, casual way Virginia throws 'laugh at my limitations' in there. But it's context, you see. Each decade has provided a different layer of perspective. Grama wrote these words in 2002. She was married in 1951. She and I talk about their love and their marriage and their equality in 2021. No – instead, see her words about their marriage for what it meant for them at the time, and then many years later.

The next generation, my mum and my dad, were not married forever. To each other, at least. That was one of the things that my grandparents' marriages held that my parents' did not: they stayed married. But there are so many more infinitesimal decisions in the older generation's relationships that ensured longevity and happiness, they are impossible to replicate. So don't. Don't try and copy any other marriage or relationship. Just check in with yourself every now and again to see if you're happier with that person than you are without. Or, alternatively, see if you can relate with Buzz when he said:

Proposing to Virginia was the best decision of my life.

This is a tricky letter to write, because this is a letter that talks about the divorces of people that are not me. Of marriages that are not mine, that ended for reasons I was not there for. And so if it seems I gloss over some of these details, it isn't because the stories are not significant – it's because the stories are owned by others.

However, my mother has written about some of those endings, so in these places I can pause a little longer. Here she is, sitting at lunch in the late 1990s.

My friend looks at me across the table.

'I can see he adores you. Is it like being a princess … being waited on hand and foot?'

'I'm a princess all right, a princess in a tower,' I want to say, but I don't. I just sit and look back at her.

'Kate, it took me two long years to leave my husband. Oh? You didn't know I was divorced? I don't claim to know everything, but I know one thing for certain. I can spot an

unhappy marriage a mile away.' She takes a sip. 'Am I wrong?'

I can't speak. My throat has shut tight. I dare not. If I do the truth will fall out of my mouth. It will be out where I have to answer to it, and I'm just not ready for that.

I cannot tell you exactly why Mum's marriages ended, but I can tell you what those endings meant for her, and when they meant something for me. Like the ending of my parents' marriage to each other. It's almost textbook-stale in its debut (the letter on the kitchen bench), the blowback (a set of pyjamas for each house, long stretches of absence, therapy – endless therapy) and the legacy (siblings, speeches and self-awareness).

Recently, together, you and I found an old diary of mine. Flicking through entries about the 1989 Moomba parade and school lunch preferences, we laughed at my terrible handwriting and questionable use of exclamation marks.

Then this, in March of 1990, at eight years old.

i now I havent writin in here for 11 days but dont blame me it's because dad's not living with us anymore oh my god! i'm seeing him on saturday i am SO NERVOS!!!!!

Now. Besides the fact that I was clearly far behind your own eight-year-old penmanship and spelling skills, it also kicked me in the guts to realise that you are about the same age now as I was when Dad left the letter on the bench. Since finding that diary, with its pillowed, lockable cover and faintly scented pages, I've watched you differently. I'm curious, knowing that as of this moment, you and I are parting at a particularly pronounced fork in the road. Yours will be an experience I haven't had – you will be living in the same house as your father for longer than I ever did. You will have an increasingly adult understanding of your parents' relationship as one whole concept, as opposed to relying on the individual mother and father to relate their own memories of how it was.

This is the first of many unshared experiences you and I will have. I'm glad for this one.

*

My mother and father were both married, and divorced, before they met one another. I know more about Mum's first husband than I know about Dad's first wife. My father has always leaned towards the discreet (or, potentially, the reticent) when it comes to his past.

Instead, Mum kept her first wedding photos in a yellowing album on the family photo shelf throughout our childhood. It's still there. Her second wedding dress, a simple brown 1970s sheath, still hangs in the back of a wardrobe. I used to play dress-ups in the strappy brown leather heels Mum wore as she spoke her vows to my father.

This ease around her past created an understanding in me that there was no shame in a legal union breaking down, particularly if it's because one's husband has been unfaithful. This is a good thing: to see your parents as fallible means you aren't so afraid to make mistakes.

Lesson #17: It is okay to fuck up.

But that marriage, the one that came before me, is her story to tell, not mine. And Dad's marriage, that one that came before Mum, is his story, not mine. However, I've been around for all the rest of their unions. The first of which, to each other, produced me and your uncle. His name is also Jim (I know – there are too many Jims in this story).

While my brother may share the name of others in this family, he is the only person in the world who understands what being a child amidst this particular set of matrimony feels like. We are four years apart in age and until recently, had never lived in the same city as adults. These, plus a hundred others, are reasons why we mightn't be close. But we are. My brother is a wonderful father, and husband and friend. He is very, very funny. And when *I* manage to make *him* laugh, I feel as if I've bottled love and pride and drunk it all up.

I don't have memories of Mum and Dad fighting. I don't have memories of them at all. Not together, anyway. There's a home video that has survived since the 1980s. Mum intended it as a 'Day in the Life' for American relatives, including Jim and Kay.

This was decades before social media. Did you know there was a time when in order to share the equivalent of a Facebook album you had to capture the imagery in hard copy and send it via International Registered Post? The twentieth century was wild, my girl.

So Mum shot the video with a groaning, creaking, plastic behemoth one day in 1989. In it, we are the perfect family. Mum, Dad, two kids. There's a dog. Cream couches. Our skin is smooth and tanned, our teeth are white. My school uniform includes a straw bowler hat. My brother is as cute and unintelligible as any gabbling three-year-old. The sun shines through the sparkling windows and Dad enters stage-left in a suit, with a knowing eye roll and charming smile. Like many children from the recorded age, I think those memories of the video have scribbled over my real ones. If I squint really hard, I wonder, maybe I can produce a real memory from the same time. Yes. It smells of lamb chops on the barbecue. There is daphne flowering at the front step. A paddling pool on dense couch grass in the back yard.

Dad moved out not long after the video was made.

Another memory that is definitely real, existing beyond photographs and home movies, is how fast I ran to Dad and how hard I hugged him after he moved out. In the week he left, I went back to that shelf of photo albums and cut out all the photos of him that I could find. Not to destroy, but to stick with Blu Tack on that secret shelf over my bed. When he arrived at the front door he knocked and waited in the doorway. Waiting. How had he morphed so quickly into someone who waited to be invited into his own home? It hurts, very much, to see a parent go from member of the household to someone who hovers at the threshold.

The Dad of my first eight years was gone and never really returned.

My father went on to have a long marriage that produced three excellent people – sisters I had always hoped for. They may have arrived a decade or two after my wishes for girl siblings began, but they were there – and still are. Their presence is something I continue to feel warm curls of gratitude for.

Another dinner party quip that I used was, 'The best marriage of my parents is the one my dad left my mum for.' I meant it with love. I was relieved that such sliced-open pain had produced something so good and solid. It turned out, eventually, it wasn't so. Twenty-odd years later the marriage ended and it was their turn for thoughts to come pouring out of their own sliced-open pain. My (now ex-) stepmother remains in our life as a wonderful mother to my three sisters. Together the four women are aunts and friends and members of our ever-expanding family group.

Dad remarried. Again. A good woman: he is happy; she is happy. I am happy for them.

*

In the years between Dad leaving Mum and her marrying her Now, her Forever Husband, she had another husband. He was a chef. He walked with a dancer's grace. He drove a Mercedes as long as a ship with deep woollen seat covers that smelt faintly of vanilla. I had lunches packed in Tupperware, straight from his restaurant's kitchen to my schoolbag. Lunchtimes as a fourteen-year-old included duck confit, risotto, steamed bok choy. Often I'd swap them for Vegemite sandwiches. The marriage ended for good one long weekend, and my brother and I walked Mum around the park while she wept. I could see how broken she was, but I also saw a light flicker at the very back of her eyes. We were back to the three of us again: Kate, Ella and Jim, a knot tied even tighter than before.

As Mum's eyes became brighter, therein shone a key lesson she taught me early on: 'It's not the end of the story. Things will get better again. I promise.'

Lesson #18: 'The End' does not mean 'The END'.

Mum fell in love for the last time with a man I'd known for a long time. A good man.

I was overseas by then, living in London. He wrote me a letter explaining their love and his intentions and how they had come about. It was so honest, so respectful. That I wasn't so floored by it shows a) how young I was, and b) that I already knew he was a good man. They married in the spring with a bagpiper striding over the park towards them and their happy brethren. Mum wore a gold-and-green dress that shimmered as she glowed.

> *Cool air, a breeze the scent of honeysuckle and hot tram dust … The oysters smell like the sea and the Champagne tingles like it. Over the rim of my glass I can see the park. I know which direction the piper will come from. There he is now, striding across the sward. No-one has noticed. His bagpipes whine like a wee tartan mozzie … The hair lifts at the nape of my neck and Ross squeezes my hand so very hard. I don't care, it's thrilling and deafening and perfect and he is surprised … just as I'd planned. I don't much like weddings, but this one is wonderful.*

My stepfather is a good man. My mother is happy; he is happy. I am happy for them.

The final wonder of my own parents' second (or third, or last) marriages is that it is no longer my responsibility to live through them. When I left home I was unfastening myself from their marriage licences, from their decrees-absolute, from their pain and from their love. I don't know what it feels like to be a child of an endlessly married couple: the dynamic is completely foreign to me. Sometimes I wonder whether leaving home gave those 'children of the forever-marrieds' the same sense of a relieved unmooring as it did me.

Lesson #19: You already have things to teach me.

So yes, being endlessly married has, until recently, remained an unfamiliar concept to me. I was out of that world for so long that now I struggle to accept my own marriage seems to have sided me with the 'other' group. For years, time spent with those whose parents were securely bound together was an exotic experience. Now with your father I am playing for Team Married.

My first head-turn of understanding at this different world is that it is not different at all.

'What's the secret to a long marriage?'

'You don't get divorced.'

I struggle with this quote. I used to love it because it instilled a power in me, a protective cloak against the blasting divorce rays of my own parent's marital collapses.

'It's okay!' I said to myself, 'All I need to do is Not Get Divorced!'

But now, I think it assumes a fault in those who have *not* had a long marriage. Those who have divorced because of abuse or trauma or – and this is just as legitimate as the former – simply not loving a person in that way anymore. Or even those who have chosen to not marry at all.

These people have not missed out on the secret to a long marriage, it is just that they have heard another, more important secret:

Lesson #20: It is okay to not be married.

And so what does all of this mean for my marriage, and (maybe, if you choose) for yours? Nothing. Your grandparents' many marriages mean nothing. Your great-grandparents' endless marriages mean nothing. Your own parents' marriage means nothing. My girl, do not feel burdened by what has come before.

There is a saying about writing: 'Some days it's easy, some days it's hard, but when you read the words back, you can't tell which day was which.' I feel the same could be said of a marriage. The more time that passes, the more the days (good, bad, or – mostly – the in-between) blend. Looking back, you don't remember the sparkles or the tears as much as feel what you have built: a union; a bond; a tied-togetherness. I'm not telling you that the troughs and peaks are forgotten; instead, I'm reassuring you that they are not all there is.

Lesson #21: What matters is the magic that can happen in the quiet spaces in between.

As I write this letter to you, daughter of mine, your father and I have been married for thirteen years. That's longer than some of my own parents' marriages, an increasingly unimportant milestone.

Tom and I were married at a winery south of Melbourne. It was a November day. In the planning, I'd had visions of a Tuscan-esque view with the late spring sun warming our backs as we said our vows looking out over the tumbling vines.

With the help of both of our families we had put together a pretty ceremony and dinner for our sixty-odd guests. It was an intimate group and because we were still young enough to believe that things needed to done A Certain Way, on the eve of the wedding the women stayed in one house and the men another.

The morning of the wedding – the early, early morning – the bride- and groom-to-be, the parents and families and friends of each party, all woke. At 3 am. To hear the clamour of the heavens and clouds and also (where did the cymbals come from?) an entire percussion section of an orchestra pit descend on the various roofs we were sleeping under.

It rained.

Oh boy, did it rain – it rained and it froze and the winery lost electricity just a few hours before the ceremony.

Luckily, no-one told me the last bit, so when I arrived, picking my way through the puddles in my white satin heels, I was smiling. A little disappointed to be wed indoors beneath the glowing green EXIT sign instead of outside by green rolling hills, but smiling nonetheless. We were with our families and our friends, and my dad walked me down the aisle, and it was a lovely day.

I look back on our wedding with a fondness for the young people we were then, as opposed to the romance of what we were celebrating. That was to come later.

Lesson #22: Don't get hung up on the wedding.
It's what comes after that counts.

I am proud of the bond Tom and I share, my girl. In just over a decade we have weathered infertility, homesickness, mental illness, cancer, death and a pandemic. There have been job moves, house moves and a baby. Over and over we have negotiated, compromised, sacrificed and lost. We have grown, too.

After all I have told you, I understand many things about marriage. I am a conjugal smart alec, smug with pain and experience. I know what it is like to have a father leave. I know what it is like to meet a step-parent and then say goodbye to one. I know what it is like to be introduced to siblings after believing no more were coming. I know what the end of a marriage looks like.

But I do not know how it feels to implicitly believe that all marriages will last forever.

What I didn't realise, until writing these letters to you, is that neither did the people in this story. The people who *were* married until the end: they did not feel the spiritual certainty I used to believe all married couples unlocked on their wedding days. Instead they just felt love, and trust and instinct – and hoped that the rest would follow. Much like your father and I. Much like Buzz and Virginia:

> *After our (1950) wedding reception, Virginia and I drove to Carmel to start our honeymoon. We had booked into a rather old fashioned inn, sort of a guest house. We had dinner in the big dining room with the other guests, none under the age of fifty, all of whom seemed amused by our age and the fact we were covered in rice and confetti. We retired to our room and quickly jumped into bed. At 3 am Virginia woke me.*
>
> *I said, 'What's wrong?' and she said,'I am hungry.'*
>
> *I lay there for a brief moment trying to figure out what she really meant. After all, I thought both of us had really enjoyed ourselves a few hours earlier. But no, she really wanted something to eat!*
>
> *I sat up in bed, turned on the light and said, 'This inn does not have room service and the nearest possible food is twelve miles away at Monterey.'*
>
> *She said she would really like a hamburger.*
>
> *I said, 'If you think I am getting dressed to drive twelve miles to Monterey, and back twelve miles, on the chance there is an all-night hamburger stand – you have the wrong impression of what to expect of your new husband. Go back to sleep!'*
>
> *She did.*

It was 1950 and these two young people had just been married. They were not expecting much. They were hopeful for what would follow. Buzz wrote about another night, a night in 1975:

On our 25th wedding anniversary I set up a black tie dinner for eight of our good friends. I was working late at the office so I changed there and Virginia was brought to the club by one of the guests. On my walk to the [dinner] I dropped into a milk bar and bought a very meagre hamburger, and slipped it into my coat pocket. At the appropriate time when the guests were toasting our twenty-five years, I took the floor and told the honeymoon story. I then produced the hamburger, maintaining Virginia had now proved she deserved it. If I had known what a great partner she was going to be, I would have driven to Monterey for that hamburger in 1950.

Because a wedding can be the beginning of many beautiful, special, painful moments. But that's what it is, just a beginning. Afterwards comes endless work to maintain, effort to grow, stubbornness to persist.

The wedding is telling your hungry bride to 'go back to sleep'. Marriage is producing a burger from your pocket, twenty-five years later.

Letter Seven

For when you're a jerk

A note on the use of the word 'jerk'. I'm not being coy, you've heard your father watch football games and your mother on work calls often enough to know all of the best profanity. So yes, I could have used others. 'Arsehat' springs to mind. 'Fuckstick' works well. But jerk is a goodie. It is not obscene, so it doesn't get blurred by outrage or offence. It's lighthearted, so it tricks people into listening, with their guard down. It almost sounds fun, until the little onomatopoeic of the 'k' in 'erk' pinches, like a needle.

In this letter, 'jerk' is not amusing, or light. In this letter, you will realise you do not want to be a jerk. In this letter, you may see that this isn't possible.

Lesson #23: If you're not already a jerk, you will become one.

You will come across a lot of people in your life who are richer or poorer than you. More or less clever. Faster on the running track or slower on the job ladder. The quickest way to become a jerk is to use these external markers as signs of whom to like, and whom to respect.

Jim shared some similar advice with Kay in response to some of her observations about her life working in Washington. About those external markers of who's 'better' or 'worse' than you:

> *You've touched on my pet hobby – valuation of humanity irrespective of class ... The more I ramble around the world, the more I see that men and women are good or bad, kind or otherwise, irrespective of that imaginary line that designates the nicer sort. Sounds trite, doesn't it? It is trite. Yet sometimes it's blamed hard to discover. I used to have an exaggerated idea of it – thought that all goodness and real value came from the back alleys and corners – sort of a diamond in the rough philosophy.*
>
> *Now I figure it's sort of a fifty-fifty proposition – you'll find about as many worthwhile personalities on the side of the 'nicer' line as on the other, and the happiness of our lives depends on whether we're lucky enough to meet 'em, and keen enough to recognize 'em when we do meet 'em.*

Does Jim sound trite? Not when we consider he was twenty-three, rolling through post-armistice France in a murk of (I assume) PTSD and homesickness. I think he's making a lot of sense. And I think Jim would approve of my belief that the fastest way for me to teach you, darling girl, how to recognise those Worthwhile Personalities, is to point out those less than worthwhile. Those ... jerks.

I'm old enough to know that regardless of what side of the imaginary line one stands on, there will be jerks around. That's been the easy part: knowing that they're there. But now, with some space and silence, I've really thought about it. And I've got the *why* as well as the what. Work has been the key to unlocking this explanation. The pay cheques I pulled across department stores, restaurants and offices also presented me with a particular perspective on jerks. How to understand them, how to avoid them, and what to do when you become one (because – as I said – you will).

Yes – I'm afraid, my girl, that your job will be where you come across the highest concentration of jerks. So I've collected three broad themes that I found across three broad industries.

Here are the jobs that taught me why people are jerks.

Hospitality

There's a lot of ignoring in hospitality. Pop on a white shirt and hold a tray and you're rendered invisible to those you're serving. Even at seventeen, I suspected this was down to those dining at the tables I was working having a chip on their shoulder. I should point out that I was a terrible waitress. The elation I experienced at the ending of each shift never outweighed the stomach-drop of fear I felt every time something went wrong.

And things going wrong generally happened as often as my shift finished: i.e. every time. The bridge between both moments could only be shortened by a smile or a thanks from one of the patrons who'd been unlucky enough to fall into my serving area. Unfortunately, those kindnesses were rarer than they should have been. Forgotten entrees or not, I'm not going to take responsibility for all the poor behaviour I was witness to across the restaurants I worked at in the late 1990s. You can call out poor service without being a jerk.

Really, I think it all comes from embarrassment. The rudest customers I served meals to were those who were uneasy about sitting where they were sitting. Maybe they hadn't been to that particular restaurant before and didn't know how to navigate the menu. Maybe their table-mate was obnoxious and their braying was carrying across the restaurant. Maybe they had ordered the wrong pasta and didn't like sun-dried tomato (this was the 1990s, after all). Looking back, whether I was ignored, dismissed or snapped at, I think most of the jerkiest patrons were holding some sort of shame.

Shame can be small and tight, held like an uncomfortable patron in a restaurant. Or it can be stretched into forever. Buzz had a birth father who was absent, and who was full of shame about it.

> *My father went out of my life when I was aged about four. As I mentioned earlier, we never heard from him again. Even his family couldn't make contact. I learned … that many years later my father's sister located him in Oklahoma. He was working on installing a telephone line. She pleaded with him to see his mother and father. He resisted at first. However, eventually he agreed to meet them but he did it in a very formal way, on the front porch of a pub. The meeting lasted about two hours and he never returned to see them again. I understand this broke the heart of my grandmother, and grandfather too. Obviously he was so embarrassed about abandoning his first wife and children that he just couldn't face his family.*

Lesson #24: Some jerks are simply embarrassed.

Retail

I worked four Christmases as one of Santa's Helpers on the Christmas floor at Myer. Visiting Myer's flagship Melbourne store at Christmas remains an annual tradition for people from all over the state, just like Virginia's experience of San Francisco's animated windows:

> *After Thanksgiving the first tinsel decorations appeared in the red and gold Woolworth's window on University Avenue. We begged to be taken to see the real windows, the animated ones in the San Francisco stores: The City of Paris, The White House and The Emporium. The theme one year was tunes from the 'Gay Nineties', a glorious epoch in the history of San Francisco. The Daring Young Man on the Flying Trapeze swung back and forth wearing colourful tights and twirling his moustache. I stood*

> *on the sidewalk, my face pressed against the icy glass, charmed by his graceful actions. Within the copper-framed window the figures of the spectators gazed up too. Wasp-waisted girls swooned, small boys ate cotton candy and the ringmaster waved his arms.*

In retail, I argue that most jerk behaviour stems from anxiety. Even though I was an *actual Christmas elf*, people were still fairly nasty. Often, I came to understand, it was because they were anxious. Anxious they'd miss their visiting slot. Anxious their child was going to have a meltdown in the hours-long queue. Anxious that when they finally got through the magical wooden doors, the Big Man wouldn't make it all worth it. When people are trying on clothes, they're anxious they won't look great. When people are perusing candles and hand cream, they're anxious they can't afford the gift. When people are visiting Father Christmas, they're worried the reality won't match the dream.

Lesson #25: Some jerks are just anxious.

Advertising

My Forever Career. The one that played the biggest part in making the professional me, me. Advertising.

Here is a quick lesson about what I've been doing for the past two decades:

My department in ad-agency life has traditionally been known as client, or account, service. Darling, account service has nothing to do with accounts in the numerical sense. Please don't let future generations think that Great-Grama Ella was an accountant. That would be offensive to all the accountants out there. While I've helped facilitate million-dollar productions, I still have to use PercentageCalculator.com to double-check sums. This is neither a lie nor an exaggeration. You were nine when you surpassed my abilities in mental arithmetic.

Nope, the hint's in 'service'. Account service is all about the *service*. Putting the money, the admin, the strategic and creative input all aside, the core focus of my job is to navigate the relationship between the Creative and the Client.

And I've worked with a lot of unkind clients. I've even worked with some jerks, and I can say after twenty-plus years of Difficult Conversations, poor professional behaviour most often sits in a place of fear. Clients who are fearful of their boss, their board or even themselves. They may be fearful of change, of sticking their heads above the parapet and jeopardising their role. The most unkind clients I've had have been those who were the most full of fear. Neither fear, nor anxiety, nor embarrassment are excuses to behave poorly. But they are explanations. And with knowledge comes power.

The first time I used this power of understanding with an enraged client, a light flicked on in my lizard brain. I'll explain, but you'll need to come down two flights of stairs to a basement edit suite that smells of expensive diffuser sticks, coffee and – faintly – the body odour of an overworked film editor. Tense advertising conversations tend to intensify in edit suites. Because:

1. It's often the first time the client has seen the 'work' (the ad) move from the page to the screen.
2. They've put a lot of money into the project.
3. The timings are always tight.
4. The stakes are high.
5. They are seated in a low sofa, knees around their ears, plied with catering and asked, six faces turned to them with bright smiles, 'Any first thoughts?'

It's a tricky time for everybody. And the most inexperienced clients are also, understandably, the most nervous.

He was a besuited man from a different generation. His watch was heavy with money and his belt tight with long lunches. He wasn't inexperienced, but he was also not listening. We delivered the idea we had sold, but it was not the execution he had expected. And I was a twenty-something woman perched on the edge of a leather couch (because I had given all the seats to the clients), trying to explain this. Spittle gathered on his lips. He gesticulated so close to my face I could see his manicure. Understanding went 'click' in my head and I realised as he shouted … this one wasn't inexperienced, but he was very afraid.

Lesson #26: Most jerks are afraid.

There's no neat ending to that interaction. He left furious in a cloud of high blood pressure and aftershave. Afterwards, I sat in the taxi waiting for my hands to stop shaking, laughing at how absurd the preceding hour had been. Since then, I've thankfully had only a few such conversations with clients. The exchanges that have produced an outcome for the better are those where we both managed to navigate each other without throwing anxiety, fear or shame into a professional conversation.

I still remember his cloudy, scared eyes, and thank him for the lesson: that understanding jerks can protect you against their spittle and waste.

It still dismays me when the person paying the bills believes it makes them more important than the one they're paying. Working in a service industry is like being dropped into a knife fight with a bottle of massage oil. You're told to avoid being stabbed – and while you're at it, try offering the person attacking you a foot rub.

Lesson #27: A service transaction doesn't dictate rank – on either side.

It's important to be kind to yourself when you inevitably act like a jerk. None of us will ever be perfect, and you are not the exception. The closest we can come to perfection is reflection, self-awareness and (if you're lucky) a little pinch of enlightenment.

Even the elders whose stories have been passed down the line have been A-Grade jerks on occasion. And those are only the instances they've committed to paper – imagine all the moments in their lives that *didn't* make it to memoir? Even Jim, whose letters can make him seem like an adventurous war hero, made some rank-pulling jerk calls.

Although in this instance, he paid for it:

I was gassed once.

It was up in the Second Argonne, toward the end of my service in France. We had captured a line of trenches, including certain dugouts that had been command posts. The Germans dug down, about 15 or 20 feet … [and] they had bunks there for the officers; telephones, communications lines, things like that. Anyway, we had captured that, and we'd been without sleep for two or three nights. My orderly and I were assigned this one little dugout, to sleep in … I went down into the place, and there were these two bunks. One, practically on the ground, just about on the floor. And the other one about three feet above it. Since I had a little trouble getting into the upper one, and since I'd ridden on tourist cars in my youth, I knew that officers should take lower berths, which were more choice.

So I chose the lower, and told my orderly to take the upper. There'd been a lot of gas used around there, and since it was heavier than air (it has to be, otherwise it floats up and doesn't do its job) the gas had soaked into the mud, and the mud had become permeated with it. It had been raining, and there was plenty of mud. The orderly and I both went sound asleep. Early in the morning, when the sun came up, and it cleared, the sun shone down the steps into the dugout and hit the ground. That volatized the gas in the mud, and it rose as high as the lower bunk, but not as high as the second bunk. I got gassed, and my orderly did not.

Which showed me the vice of trying to be snooty and choose the best accommodations.

Lesson #28: Sometimes, let someone else pick the first bunk.

This is not a letter of repression. I'm not telling you to quash your rage, or ignore your hurt. I am not telling you to avoid being embarrassed, anxious or afraid. I acknowledge that all of these emotions are real. Sometimes they're valid, sometimes they're *warranted*. Often, they're forgivable. And they are always human. You can be fallible, my girl. You can be all of these boring, brutish things, as long as you try and temper them with kindness.

Back in France, Jim had an experience with a general who didn't allow rank to interfere with practicality – and kindness.

[After arriving in Le Mans] I went to my new Colonel immediately, and I said, 'Where's my horse?'

He said, 'Well, a funny thing happened about that horse, Quinby. We got her back to the regiment all right, and she came back here with us. But it appears you've been outranked. The lieutenant colonel, who's the adjutant to the brigadier, liked that horse, so he grabbed her and is now using her for himself.'

So I rather forced my way in to see the general. I put on this big act, about Betty. How I loved her, what she had done when I was wounded, and just generally hammed it up.

So he finally interrupted me and said, 'Stop it, stop it. I get the point.' And he grabbed a piece of paper, wrote something, and said, 'Here, take this to the colonel. That's all.'

So I thanked him and went out the door. When I looked at the paper, it said, 'Give this man his horse.' That simple and that direct.

So I looked around until I saw the colonel riding my horse. I went up to him and saluted, and handed him this paper. He was a good Joe. He read the paper, stuffed it in his pocket, got off my horse, and said 'Can you ride this horse bare-back?'

I said, 'Yessir.'

Then he said, 'The reason I ask is that this saddle is my property.'

So he took the saddle off, and the last I saw of him he was trudging back towards his headquarters carrying his saddle. I got on Betty, and she and I went back to the headquarters of the regiment.

It can be hard to be kind to people when they're waving a dagger at you. You don't need to rub their feet, but you can try and remember that they're juggling embarrassment, anxiety or fear. None of these are excuses, but they're explanations. And explanations that lead you to knowledge can also lead you to understanding. It might be too late to help that diner, that shopper, or that client – but it's not too late to help yourself.

And this is where we move to me and some of the times *I've* been a jerk.

My girl, these letters have forced me back into the shaded parts of my diaries and memory and … ouch. It will not surprise you to hear that I have been a jerk often, persistently, brilliantly.

When I was fourteen I dumped a sweet boy with no notice or explanation. I literally danced a jig of heady relief under the clocks of Flinders Street Station. Yet when I looked up he hadn't stepped onto his departing tram. Instead, he was standing still, watching me, eyes round with sadness.

I'd been so unsure about the act of ending a relationship that I bumbled through the process, ashamed at my naivety.

My embarrassment made me a jerk.

My first bout of true, crippling anxiety broke out during a particularly hard London winter, and it rendered me socially selfish and emotionally incapable. I was a burden to my colleagues, friends and flatmates. I was rolling between rosé and reclusion, ignoring phone calls and forgetting dinner dates.

My anxiety made me a jerk.

Around the same time, I nearly lost your father through fear. I was not kind to him, I was not kind to the lover I was leaving – and I was certainly not kind to myself. My ego will tell you it's because I'd sensed that I had found a lifelong love at an inconveniently young age. My conscience will tell you that I was simply scared of what I was leaving and what I was running towards.

My fear made me a jerk.

Lesson #29: Don't let self-awareness turn into self-flagellation.

I feel relieved that I moved through a lot of this poor behaviour when I was so young. Twenty-one, twenty-two, a basic baby ricocheting between friends and jobs and boys and hearts and not doing a very good job with any of them. Luckily my youth cushioned me from being too mean: I just didn't know enough to be truly cruel. The older you get, the more brutal you can become. You know too much; you know how to let the blows land so they hurt.

Lesson #30: If you're young, forgive yourself. If you're not, stop.

The older you get, the more likely you are to use your words as your weapon. The most jerky things one does often include words. Cruel words. Words that fly out of your mouth before you've had a chance to taste how terrible they are. Be very, very careful about what you say when you're wild, sad or just bored. Be careful about words said to someone's face, but be just as careful about those spoken behind their back.

Just. Be. Careful.

Do not think that what you say will disappear, just because you will want them to afterwards. Regret does not undo malice. The only way to cleanse a relationship from nasty words is with love, apology, good intention and time. Yet even then, the stain of what was said can remain.

Lesson #31: Angry words come from sad people.

Cruel words are slivers of shrapnel embedded in the body of the person you threw them at. Every person in your family carries a wound from a word thrown in anger, including me. Some have submitted to an entire arsenal. Do you remember Jim's shrapnel scar, the one Virginia was fascinated by?

Fourteen years earlier he lay on a bed in a hospital in London, where two doctors looked at an X-ray and said to Jim:

> *'What do you think we ought to do?'*
>
> *And I said, 'You're asking me? Well, heavens, what would you do if it was your carcass?'*
>
> *And they said that they'd talked that over, and they thought they'd prefer to leave the shrapnel pieces there. The reason was that this was before the invention of antibiotic drugs, and whenever they mentioned an operation that might lay open the cavity above the lung, they talked about pneumonia, and bowed sadly, because there was no cure, and the rate of fatality was great.*
>
> *So I said okay, and they left them there.*
>
> *[Sixty-seven years later] I still have them in there, although they have given me no pain or trouble since.*

Don't be one of those people who has caused that kind of leaden barrage. A body will heal, and grow around the scar, but the metal will remain.

Lesson #32: Use your words as if they will last forever.

You may think it unfair of me to finish a letter filled with faults with a request to be better. A request to be gracious. A request to be kind.

But I don't have much concern about seeking this from you, darling. You have come from a family where kindness is inherent.

Don't misunderstand this; we are not an angelic group. Nor are we saccharine or sappy. If this family is a seasoning, our kindness is a compound: we cut any sweetness with a mix of bitter, sour and salty. Like anything true in this world, our kindness is multidimensional, with a dark and light side. But this is a good thing – it means our kindness is genuine. Our kindness is true.

There is a certain look in someone's eye when they realise that you are only being kind to them because you want something. It's horrible. It's like they've found you out. Don't get me wrong, it's perfectly acceptable to use kindness as a means to an end – but you must also use it when there's no end at all. Because there lies a very powerful magic in handing over a small envelope of kindness to someone who can do absolutely nothing for you in return.

It's a brave author who disagrees with Roald Dahl, but here it goes. He once said, 'Throw kindness around like confetti'.

I don't subscribe to the confetti approach. Throwing it around haphazardly, watching it float and drift away, doesn't seem to respect kindness for what it really is. Which is, the opportunity to change the programming of someone's brain.

You have that power! This is not a time for confetti-chucking!

No.

I say: present kindness in little boxes, head bowed. Slide kindness into thick creamy envelopes, with expensive-tasting glue. Post kindness, over and over, in a mail subscription service. Do it mindfully, earnestly, with eye contact and sincerity. If delivered with the right intent, kindness is never weak. Kindness is not bleach. Kindness doesn't delete other attributes it's paired with. You can be kind *and* strong. Kind *and* clever.

Lesson #33: Try to be kind.

Letter Eight

Tastes

When you die slowly, it is said your senses depart one by one. Taste, smell, touch and sound. They are guests leaving a party, waving farewells and disappearing into the dark.

One of the first senses to withdraw is taste. Which is such a pity, for me, because I love to eat. Luckily, I also love to read about eating and, most fortunately, our family loves to write about it. Of all the words they have shared, food has attracted some of the most loving of descriptions.

Because this family really loves food. When Grama began her four years at college in 1944, lunch was often an extended affair:

> *'Lucy and John's' was one of our favourite restaurants, though with gas rationing I can't remember how we got up to Foothill Boulevard [from college]. But we'd arrive, over a dozen girls to a table, and begin prolonged discussions of what to order from the extensive menu. Huge plates of spaghetti were only thirty cents. A five-course dinner of soup, salad, antipasto, spaghetti and ravioli, chicken or steak, dessert, coffee, tea, milk or buttermilk – cost two dollars. A side order of french fries was fifteen cents. Coffee was five cents a cup and a basket of their wonderful*

garlic bread was twenty-five cents. We'd wolf down our food in about fifteen minutes then spend half an hour settling the account.

'Who had the garlic bread?'

'I didn't order the salad!'

'You had two cups of coffee.'

Lesson #34: As soon as you can afford to, shout the meal.

I am inviting you to read a meal with me. It's going to be wonderfully chaotic, which is just the way this family likes to eat. There will be crispy syllables, juicy verses and a sprinkled seasoning of punctuation. Some dishes you've already eaten dozens of times. Others, you won't have known could be eaten at all.

Take, for instance, a lunch Buzz shared with colleagues during a visit to Yemen in the 1960s. It was at the house of a customer of his, and at the time the only way to visit the town 'was to drive along the beach at low tide'.

They had a lunch for us. We were all sitting on the floor using our left hand to eat, as is the custom. They were all sitting around with bands of bullets slung across their chests and pistols and knives in their belts. At first I thought they were just for decoration but they seemed to be prepared to attack at any time. They did have a sense of humour though because they maintained that since lamb was what we were eating, and as I was the honoured guest, I would have the sheep's eye. Well, have you ever tried to eat a sheep's eye? They're so tough you can't bite it in half and it's too big to swallow whole.

I have not eaten a sheep's eye, but I have dissected one in science class and I can confirm: Buzz was correct.

We have a family tradition of discussing the next meal as we commence the current one. Even our traditional American

Christmas lunch with turkey, stuffing, mashed potato, gravy, cornbread, pumpkin pie and 'hard sauce' will end with 'What are we having for dinner?'

That dinner then finishes with 'What time is breakfast?'

Yet this time, as we read a whole meal together, we'll be dining on dishes that stretch over breakfast, lunch, dinner and one hundred years in between. So, pull up a chair. Sit here, next to me. Sweep the crumbs from the embroidered linen placemats. Do you like the violets? Yes, I know they're sitting in a wine bottle, but today, it's being used as a vase. I hope you're hungry.

*

It's best to start with breakfast, which in this family must include waffles. Before they emigrated permanently to Australia in 1969, Buzz, Virginia and their children were as American as Route 66 and 'Lucy and John's'. And even after then, many of this family's traditions, recipes and family rhythms remain bedded in the USA.

Of all the waffles we have made over the years, my brother, Jim may have put away the most. Virginia tells of the mountains she cooked for him during long summers at the surf lifesaving club, where he was living every teenager's dream. I expect Jim needed all of the breakfast fuel he could wolf.

Now. I know you understand how special our family yeast waffle recipe is – but you must ensure *others* know too. Because these are not some sugary confection bought pre-cooked and frozen. These are waffles that require planning, an overnight proofing and all the patience a crispy-on-the-outside, fluffy-on-the-inside breakfast requires. For decades Virginia was the keeper of the waffle iron for our family:

> *Our family yeast waffle recipe has come a long way from 19th century (or earlier) Maryland, USA to Point Lonsdale, Australia.*

During the summers when Jim was at the Surf Club he enjoyed waffles many mornings. He'd always ask me if it was OK. Was that out of consideration? Or was it to make sure I set enough yeast to rise the night before? I loved feeding him, his mates, his girlfriends and once, during Bronze Camp, even his coach.

Batter ingredients
2 cups milk, lukewarm
1 packet dry yeast (approx 2 ¼ teaspoons)
1 tablespoon sugar
½ teaspoon salt
2 cups plain flour
⅓ cup melted shortening
¼ teaspoon baking soda dissolved in a little hot water
2 eggs
(You're going to need a large, four-sectioned American-style waffle iron)

In recent years, my mother Kate has taken up the mantle:

Method
The night before, mix together the milk, yeast, sugar, salt and flour and let rise overnight in a covered bowl. In the morning add melted shortening, baking soda in water and the two egg-yolks and whites, beaten separately. Gently fold together (don't over-blend) and tip the batter into a pouring jug. When the waffle iron is really hot, pour a generous blob into the centre, covering about half of the iron. Let it cook until properly golden brown and crispy. Undercooked, flabby waffles are awful.

Lesson #35: Butter <u>before</u> syrup.

My waffle memories begin much earlier, when I was about six and my brother was only two. The pair of us would sit at Shenzi's kitchen table, eyeing the waffle iron like hawks. We had a rule that whoever spied the iron's light blink on to red, received the first waffle from that batch. The light had no sound to accompany it, so a vigilant watch was needed.

Blink.

A chorus – 'It's on!'

And here it is. A golden square handed across the table by Grama, speared on the end of a fork, piping hot and smelling of nutty yeast and sweetness. You'll have to transfer it from her fork to your plate without burning your fingers. Butter goes on first, melting quickly into the deep squares. Then (proper) Canadian maple syrup, which in my childhood was as rare as saffron and even more expensive. Watch it drip from the nozzle to your plate In. Achingly. Slow. Motion.

Eat with crispy American-style bacon and repeat until you can no longer feel your toes.

While we're eating our waffles, we'll ask one another, 'What's for lunch?'

The answer today is: a proper English roast.

We are moving from American fare to British, which is what Jim did in 1918 as the US Army sailed him from the States to Europe. He was not pleased with the food he received in the United Kingdom. In one of his letters to Kay, he said, 'You have no idea what a problem the eats question is over here.'

I too had been warned of British fare, before I set off for the (other) motherland. Instead, I found most food in London to be fresh, good and – thankfully – cheap.

There were, however, moments when the 'eats question' got the better of me, such as when I dined in my first greasy English pub. I was delighted to see 'Scampi' on the menu – and so cheap, too! Which was lucky, given my minimum wage salary. I was young, naive, and my mother had been married to that chef for a few years. So to me, scampi was a small lobster sold at great expense in Australia; its delicate flesh often served in a buttery sauce atop pasta. I had eaten scampi exactly once in my life and remembered every bite.

The scampi at the Lord John Russell in Holborn were deep-fried nuggets of some indistinguishably fish-flavoured protein. No wonder I received change from a fiver.

Given my mother's side of the family, I had a childhood flavoured with American food. Which meant my experience in England was even more foreign, because dishes that most of my Australian compatriots would see as 'old-fashioned', came to me as delightfully new.

This confusion will not be a problem for you, as your father is a Brit, born and bred. As a toddler, Tom famously snacked on 'a pork pie and a bottle of cold tea', and if that isn't the most English thing you've ever heard, I'll eat my (pork-pie) hat.

The first pork pie I ever ate was a Marks & Spencer version, the gelatinous meat set in a sweet hot-water-crust pastry. I think I was too stunned by the audacity of the dish itself to balk at the ingredients. Fat and meat, gelatine and pastry. I revelled in the unapologetic history of it all. Delicious.

The British gastronomic adventures continued. Another extraordinary combination of ingredients is blood sausage. My inaugural experience of Burns Night was at my first 'proper job' in London after arriving in the preceding June. Marked on January 25, the night celebrates the birthdate of Scotland's best-known poet, Robert Burns. I stood in the basement kitchen of the advertising agency on a cold winter's eve and listened to a Scot recite Burns' poem 'Address to a Haggis'. It was dramatic, unfamiliar and made me feel intensely how far from Melbourne I was. Afterwards we toasted with whisky and the aforementioned haggis. My first tastes of both, and both revolting. I loved it.

Lesson #36: Taste anything, everything, once.

I'll apologise in advance to the Scots reading this letter, for Jim really puts the boot into your cuisine (and the accent – ahem):

> *On the British Isles you have to have a meat card to get anything except eggs. The Scotch waitress came to our table and said 'Ah weel! Ah can gie ye soup and Ah can gie ye ham an' eggs wi'oot the ham, but Ah can na gie the one we the ither. Ah, tak em awa doon staihs an gie 'em a dinnah.' And she did but we made the mistake of taking the soup.*

Seeing as this was 1918, and the Scots were battling the Spanish Flu, the tightening of food rationing and a little thing like a world war – I'm sure they weren't too fussed about laying on a spread for some American officers.

Needless to say, Jim did not like the soup.

Scampi-gate aside, everything I ate in British pubs was a divine exercise in comfort food on crack. Pork scratchings: crispy fat in a bag? Sign me up! Yorkshire puddings: golden boats holding glossy gravy – yes please! In fact, the whole roast lunch shebang. Oh my. Eating a Sunday roast behind fogged-up pub windows is a midwinter English delight.

Lesson #37: Have Sunday lunch.

My Sunday roast preference starts with lamb. Beef is second choice, then pork, and then – if pressed – the chicken comes last. There's a pecking order ('scuse the pun) of meats which puts me at odds with my ancestors. In particular, Jim.

Which brings us back to lunch, where we will have roast chicken. For two reasons: a train filled with coffee, and a French orphan called Madeleina.

In 1902, Jim's parents migrated from the east to the west of the United States. Jim was seven years old and rode in the upper berth of the tourist car, so that 'every time we went around a curve the baggage fell over on me'.

> *We came west by railroad, by way of the Great Northern. In those days, there were two kinds of sleeping cars: the Pullman, which was for fancy and elite people; and the tourist car, which was for the likes of us … At the end of the car, there was a big stove, with a scuttle of coal. The passengers had brought food, and they made coffee and cooked on the stove. The people on the car took turns at it, so there was a big kettle of coffee going all the time. My mother fixed cold roast chicken; she had dozens of them in her great big suitcases. Whole chickens, roasted ahead of time, so that she just warmed them up.*

Sixteen years later Jim travelled from the West Coast of the States to France via train, ship and horse. In August 1918, he was billeted in a French village. While he and his fellow officers waited ('Our fighting history has not yet begun but we have hopes') they befriended some locals.

There was his landlady, Madame Delampre:

> *The Madame is a fat lady with twinkling eyes who, whenever she gets in the slightest degree 'lit' insists on a vivid description of the time she visited Paris to see the Exposition. It would be all right with me if she didn't persist in showing us by personal demonstration just how the heavy traffic goes in the city. 'Beaucoup – Beaucoup – Beauuuuu – coup de fiacres!'*
>
> *Then she illustrates and bang goes some furniture.*
>
> *Oh well, I don't care. It's her house.*

And there was Madeleina.

> *Madeleina – I told you about her, didn't I – the little orphan girl across the street? – staked us to a party last evening. Brought us*

a bottle of wine and some cookies she had made. Helped us drink the wine, too, even if she is only seven years old …

La Petite Madeleina gave a chicken dinner the night before we left, and ran after me down the road in the morning to give me a bottle of white wine for my saddle bags. The chicken dinner was fine, although the Capt. (who is somewhat sensitive) was taken aback at the French custom of cooking the head and feet of the fowl along with the rest of it. He finally conceded that we were lucky to find no feathers in the dish.

Lesson #38: The meal is often made by the company.

And so, as a toast to Jim and Madame and little orphan Madeleina, we will have roast chicken and white wine for lunch. (Let's try to keep the children from the wine, though …)

*

Lunch is over. It's time for dinner. And because I love to eat in a way that encourages indecision and rewards thievery, we'll consider a meal served tapas-style with as many different dishes as possible.

Once, after being starstruck by Jennifer Ehle at the Old Vic, your father and I were starving. It was 11 pm. We had been dating each other for over a year at this point, and Tom knew me well enough to note the signs that I was becoming hungry and cross. In the back streets of Southwark, I edged close to weeping in irritation as Tom passed all the 'post-theatre' touristy restaurants. Places that I, a relatively new Londoner, would've entered out of impatience and greed.

But he pushed me on, past the council estates, under the bridge, through the construction site, to a little tapas bar glowing in the black. It was worth it. A restaurant filled with a haze of smoke and cooking oil, and staffed by young Spanish boys with long eyelashes and no English. We ate oily cheesy meaty dishes and drank Spanish beer, and I was glad he'd made us keep walking.

Lesson #39: The best food is worth going further for.

No smoke or oil, but another London meal we may want to consider for our dinner sits at the other end of the scale – Gordon Ramsey's flagship restaurant in South London. It was still the mid-2000s and Ramsey was at the peak of his TV fame, and also of his cooking fame.

Tom's grandmother was generously hosting the whole family (and one Australian interloper – hi). The dining room was a deceptively modest space, with more staff than diners. At twenty-four years old, it was the most special restaurant I'd ever set foot in. The food was excellent, but it was the experience that made me feel exultant. Every dish that was served was accompanied by a flock of waitstaff dressed in black, gathering around the table like regal birds. They simultaneously alighted at each person's shoulder, carefully spooning sauce from a silver jug with a delicate little ladle, all the while describing the dish before us in Continental murmurings. I was in awe of the entire evening, and especially so that I had been included in this family occasion. I still remember how special it made me feel.

Lesson #40: Never forget what special feels like.

You don't need to have dined in a Michelin-starred restaurant to realise that there is a chemical reaction that occurs on your tastebuds when you eat food in a different time zone. Tom and I went to Bali in 2011 to forget that we hadn't managed to have any children. We had been married for less than a year and I was due to start IVF on returning. We stayed in a little villa in Petitenget, where we awoke each morning to frangipani lying confettied and browning across the kikuyu grass, as if we had missed an overnight wedding party.

In Bali, we ate at all the restaurants people told us to eat at. Good food, served by tanned Australians with lots of teeth and the air of people who had something to escape from. This corner of the island felt like Byron Bay and smelt like clove cigarettes. Towards the end of the trip, we came upon a side-of-the-road *warung* with caustic fluorescent lighting and a sliced oil-drum barbecue billowing smoke onto the road. The food was prepped and cooked before us, and the service was friendly, in a distracted way. But it was certainly worth waiting for. The dishes were fresh, moreish and unexpected – a boon after nights of same-same menus. We ate whole red snapper in coconut husk, and satay with generous hocks of ginger and peanuts. And *kangkung tumis terasi*: water spinach liberally tossed in coconut oil and shrimp paste. A dish so fresh, yet so unfamiliar, that I thought about it all the next day. We returned for dinner that night.

Lesson #41: Don't be afraid to repeat what's good.

Dinner's choices have ranged between tapas, Michelin-starred theatre and a roadside Balinese *warung*. But you can't decide yet. Because we're off to Paris. My first visit to the city with your father ended up at a crooked little restaurant in the back streets of Le Marais. I was a novice at the snails Tom ordered, but was more intimidated by the curved serving implements than the crustaceans themselves. I clinked the tongs curiously while we waited for the wine to be poured.

Virginia ate snails in France, too. In France, and in Ghana:

> *[My friend] Augie was from Kumasi, up-country, and on one shopping expedition found some of her favourite delicacies, land snails with conical shells the size of a fist. The woman in the stall wrapped them loosely in newspaper and put them in my basket.*

As we walked on through the market I felt something on my wrist. Much to Augie's delight a snail was tentatively feeling its way out of the basket, leaving a slimy trail across my wrist and up my arm.

While a gastropod bangle seems attractive enough a proposition, I think I'm relieved that their Parisian counterparts remained on their plate.

Virginia's visit to Paris in the 1960s included a meal just as traditional as snails:

On our last night in Paris … we strolled around the cobblestoned square below Sacré-Cœur, fascinated by the work of the various painters. Jim bought a bunch of violets from an old woman and we went to a tiny bistro for dinner. Only six or seven tables and a piano. I stuck my violets in the top of the wine bottle and spent the evening singing and devouring onion soup, crusty bread, salad, Camembert and Brie, then back to the hotel through sparkling Paris.

As romantic as this evening sounds, I'll still argue that while Paris has snails, Italy has everything, and my meals in *that* country sit as some of my favourite. My grandparents' picnic beneath the ancient arches of an olive grove in Tivoli should seal this for you:

In Tivoli … we strolled around the Villa d'Este with its witty fountains and cascades of wisteria against warm stone walls. Later we found the perfect place for a picnic in an old olive grove and sprawled among the wildflowers, whittling off pieces of bread and cheese, sipping wine and dribbling blood-orange juice off our chins.

There was one particular dinner that I will put forward, as argument and plea to convince you that our final meal should rest with the Italians.

This dinner is the closest we'll come to that five-course 'Lucy and John's' menu Virginia touched on. Yet rather than hiking up a hill in the middle of a wartime gas shortage, Tom and I only had to amble from our villa through the Puglian olive groves to the dining area of the *masseria* in which we were staying.

Sitting in the white-blue of Borgo San Marco's courtyard, we ate crispy fava beans and sipped a G&T with a satisfying clout. Our dusky-voiced chef summoned us to the verandah, and we sat down by the cool green blanket of grass and embarked on dinner. It feels wanting, to describe it as dinner. We embarked on *il viaggio.*

We began with what can only be described as my mother's very excellent puttanesca, but rather than being served with pasta, the sauce was wrapped in crumbling folds of puffed pastry. Next, sweet mussels shared their shells with creamy risotto, hidden among lush blocks of sliced potatoes. Third course was a plate of tiny octopus sitting in tomatoey jewels of pasta. Red wine was poured from a white china pig. No-one spoke English, so the chatter around us sounded like music. Our main was a glistening, whole sea bass – fresh, unadorned and fleshily delicious. We finished with stone fruit, sweet like a punch-in-the-mouth after eating imports for months.

After glasses of rosé, home in the late-night cool of our terrace, Tom and I doubled back to the main house and snuck in a quiet midnight swim. We shared the pool with nothing but a few floating olive leaves and one enormous green frog, slowly breaststroking lengths beside us. Water sounds different under stars.

Lesson #42: Swim at night, whenever you can.

Yes. I think this is where we'll settle for our dinner. Frog not included.

Letter Nine

Run away

For many years, including all of the time I was actually in the city, I believed London was a place that I had run towards. Because it was home to a man that I had run to be with. However looking back, I now realise London was more about what I was leaving behind.

And this is what travel is. This is what 'leaving yourself behind' is. This is what bedding down in a foreign city, surrounded by the alien hints and subtleties and winks and a new address, is all about.

No matter what you think you've arrived for, the bubble of being 'Other' will teach you – quickly or eventually – that your arrival was much more about the departure than what preceded it. This is why moving to London on nothing more than a fortnight's love affair and a penchant for Richard Curtis films was the best decision I ever made. It was the hardest thing I ever did, and one of the silliest, but the move also sculpted more of my self than any other experience I had, for years before, and after.

Lesson #43: Live away from home.
Live as far away as you can get.

In 2003 I was twenty-one, and knew everything. I had visited destinations before I moved to live overseas, but I'd never travelled, only holidayed. I was ready to live away. It was my time.

'How lucky for me,' I thought, as I booked my one-way ticket. 'How lucky that I already know *all* the things!'

Twenty-one and knowing all the things: what a heady, ripe time to fall in love. Six months before I flew to London, Christmastime brought an old crush back to Melbourne for the festive season. Of course, he was older than before, but he was also more tangible, and (thrillingly, for me) paying attention. It was a flushed love affair of two entire weeks, bookended by kisses in summer-humid nightgardens with cigarette mouths. He flew home to London and left me with a heart-wrenching crush and an unwashed T-shirt, which I inhaled daily, like an addict blissful in freefall.

Half a year later, with countless emails but only one night together between us, I moved to London to live out my days with my One True Love.

Did I mention, I knew all the things?

In two weeks I had fallen for a boy with a crooked smile, but I had been falling for London for years.

Looking at the family history, England was always going to go one of two ways for me. Grama loves England. Great-Grampa, not so much. Luckily for me, I received my gift from the former. Maybe I'm genetically predisposed to sarcasm, and pubs with hops hanging in boughs over the bar, and street lamps lighting walls older than my city. And while he mightn't have been London's biggest fan, Jim's descriptions of the city in 1918 do suggest some degree of affection:

Yours truly has been busily engaged in exploring the highways and byways of 'Lunnon', not to mention the side-lights and the shadows. I can balance a monocle and a cigarette holder in an otherwise innocent face, and have learned to argue in a high tone of voice with the fruiterer as to whether grapes should sell for two bob sixpence ha-penny, or for a straight 'arf crown. I have been to two or three dances, and can make a fair guess at what an English girl means when she says 'Re-a-ally', or 'Raw-THER'.

And the longer I stay here, the more I admire the French nation.

Great-Grampa's admonishment of my adopted city might have something to do with the fact that he spent much of his London time in a hospital for returned servicemen, where he was recovering from being blown up by artillery in Belgium. Before he got to see the 'side-lights and shadows', Jim was confined to a hospital in Regent's Park:

[After] they operated on me over in France, [they] sent me to London. At this hospital I have every comfort I could ask – except the absence of nice old ladies who come around to visit.

Within a few days I shall get up and take a slant at London.

My first slant at London was from far above, jetting in on June 21, 2003. I flew on an aeroplane whose overhead lockers burst open every time we landed, like enormous plastic party poppers. It would have felt celebratory if I wasn't so concerned I was going to die.

Virginia, on the other hand, first sighted England from the sea, forty-two years after her father and forty-three years before me. She was rather pregnant with her third child, and nearing the end of the Grand Tour that she and Buzz had begun in Singapore.

We left on the Paris–Calais train, boarded the Calais–Dover steamer at four in the afternoon, and I threw up about four-thirty. Once I'd accomplished that I felt quite alright. But when the cliffs of Dover came in sight I was too emotional to feel sick. After the exotic places we'd seen, it was good to be in a place that was so familiar, though neither of us had ever been there.

Virginia and Buzz felt an immediate familiarity with the United Kingdom. I expected the same – same language, same everything, right? But it was all new and upside down.

I had no idea how topsy-turvy my life was about to get.

I arrived in a heatwave and had never seen contrails like those that webbed over my new city. They laced and branched in a canopy of welcome, as my love and I flung ourselves back onto the grass of Regent's Park, our lips already swollen from kissing.

Day two introduced a heady tar-scent that pumped up from the streets, in weather the city was not built to withstand. My neck was on a swivel as I encountered every normal thing with abnormal levels of fascination.

You're never more keenly aware of how foreign a foreign city can feel when you haven't anticipated it. Before the sun had set on my first week in London I had the strange sense of something peeling away in my chest. It was the feeling of being untethered. I was loose, floating above every day I'd lived before, adrift on a current in the wrong hemisphere. It was the feeling of not knowing what was going to come next.

Lesson #44: The absence of familiarity is especially acute when you have been expecting the opposite.

Nevertheless, I fell for it all. The monocles, the cigarette holders and the 'rawTHERs'. I fell for the heady breathlessness of living in a completely different place, and I began to fall for the knowledge that no-one knew who, or why, I was.

When I told my father I was moving to London to live with a boy he hadn't yet met (and I really only had just met myself) I was shot with an electric thrill on seeing his reaction. His surprise showed me I was doing something a little wild, a tad reckless … But I was also entirely certain that this was the man I was going to spend the rest of my life with. My certainty – no matter how ill-placed, gave me a feeling of complete surety that I don't think I've ever had again. Did I mention I knew all the things?

My head spun with the romance of it all. When that man left Melbourne, left me inhaling his T-shirt, I bought the first of a hundred international phone cards and leaped hook, line and love into the drama and magic of the first-ever Love Story I'd had the chance to star in.

January, February, March – the most chaste of love affairs: lengthy phone conversations (landlines only) and endless emails. What timing – I had managed to have a long-distance love affair in the dying hours of the pre-tech age, where social media and wifi did not exist. Letters in envelopes, postcards in boxes; the dragging analogue delay added to the drama. We were in love with being in love and by April I had booked my ticket and he'd arranged a flat. Our flat. To live in together.

Did I mention the sum total of two weeks? Did I mention I knew all the things? Did I mention that I'd never left home and I'd never paid a utilities bill and I'd never been in love like I was at that very moment?

This isn't a tale of warning, my darling girl. I enjoyed every minute and I hope you will have adventures just as safe and lovely as I did. But – holy cow! – moving 16,000 kilometres on a wing and a snog was such an incandescently reckless thing to do. I'm so grateful I did. I'm grateful my family didn't stop me, and I'm grateful that the man on the other end of the very (very) long flight was kind (if a little ill-equipped) to a neurotic 21-year-old fronting up with visions of domestic perfection.

Lesson #45: Try and do your stupid things with kind people.

I wasn't completely naive. I knew what it was like to have my heart broken, what it was like to be left by a parent, and what it was like to go through loss and sadness and pain. But I didn't know how to live with someone who wasn't genetically obligated to care for me. And I didn't know how to change a lightbulb. As 2003 drew into a northern autumn and then a brutal winter, I began to think … maybe, maybe I don't know *all* the things?

But by then, it was too late. London had me.

*

London is a magical city. There's nothing I can tell you about it that hasn't been written a thousand times over. And while I can't tell you about London, I can tell you about *our* London: mine, and that of those who travelled before me.

My first London was a Top Floor Flat on Delancey Street in Camden. It was opposite a Portuguese deli that I was surprised to find also sold booze. Specifically, £3 bottles of red that tasted better than anything I'd been able to afford in the pub back home. Flaky empanadas. Cigarettes in packs of ten. Homemade custard tarts.

The flat was up innumerable flights of stairs that took me past doors in a way that made it feel oddly as if I was in someone else's house. Then I realised: it was someone else's house. Well, at least it used to be. And we were living in the servant's quarters up the top. In London, few buildings exist that haven't held a hundred souls before you.

We had a pull-down ladder that took us to the flat roof where we sat in the evenings, the warmth of the sun still captured and glowing in the black tar under our bums. We drank beer and smoked cigarettes and watched those contrails again, fading from white to orange to grey in the late setting sun. The chimney pots were round and friendly. We shagged on the roof and hoped others couldn't see.

Lesson #46: When you have sex on a roof, people can probably see.

My second London was a basement flat under a red-bricked pile behind Marylebone Station. It was the one with the pinboard from Melbourne. There wasn't anything else on the walls, so I set to dressing them on my minimum wage. In the studio at work there were enormous glossy books filled with photographers' folios. I found a bunch I liked and heaved them onto the colour photocopier, sliding the A1 prints off the machine and into a case to get them home on the bus without crumpling them. With Blu Tack and a ruler, my room was dressed.

Just as I had never lived in the eaves of a house before, I'd also never lived in the basement either. The room had been painted a deep purple by some tenant past and I stuck as many things on the wall as I could to avoid the creeping feeling that I was sleeping amid an enormous bruise. But I was bruised, then. That London, that summer, I hurt hard and deep.

I may have fallen from a Top Floor Flat to a contused room in a basement, but that room, around the corner from Madame Tussaud's waxworks and the Sea Shell chippie, was the place where I was forced to find a new London, alone. If I'd known Jim had lived so close (but nearly ninety years far-away), then maybe I would not have felt so lonely:

> *On my way back … I dropped in at Madame Tussaud's Waxwork display. Same as the Eden Museé in New York. Some very lifelike figures – Chamber of Horrors, etc. Also a tearoom. I'm afraid I'm getting the tea habit. I draw the line, though, at drinking tea in the theater. They come around at the matinee – right in the middle of an act, and serve tea. At the movies, too – anywhere – 4.30 means tea. Talk about the drink habit!*

The three girls I shared the basement flat with drank tea. They drank tea and sat on the couch watching the tiny telly sitting at a 180 degree tilt atop a wooden dining chair. I don't think they liked me very much. Looking back, I am not surprised.

I was confused and selfish and busy leaving the man I had been planning to spend the rest of my life with. And so every night I stomped my Topshop-cowboy boots across the parquet flooring, full of booze and bravado. I was extremely thin and really very sad. The basement flat was where I decided not to escape the broken relationship and flee back to Melbourne, no matter how much I was crying at night.

If I kept drinking, working, and flirting with the man at work with the blue, blue eyes, then maybe I'd forget how far my first year in London had strayed from my plan.

I was twenty-three and I really knew nothing at all.

In that second year of London I was alone in the city but starting to see things in a more sparkly way. My gloom was lifting and I was laughing more. Photos show me laughing a lot, actually. I was all teeth, and sex. My first spike of homesickness had faded, and I'd even had a flying trip back to Australia to remind myself of the things I missed. (Electric-blue light. Petrichor. Bindies. Cicadas. Molten steering wheels.) What that trip home also did was crack the rose-coloured lens I'd applied to Melbourne in my first year away. All the things I hadn't missed were still there. (A small town where everyone knows your name. Terrible newspapers. An empty bed. Molten steering wheels.) I was simultaneously relieved and immediately homesick to return to a long January of snow, fog and dark afternoons.

Lesson #47: You can be happy and sad at the same time.

In the summer of 2004 I stopped seeing the crooked-smiled man I'd moved to England to love. I was also trying rather hard to stop seeing a blue-eyed Englishman who had made things quite a bit more complicated than I had planned for.

When you are freshly single and trying hard to remain so, you tend to travel further for less, more often. Weekends can be especially lonely, so when people ask you to 'Come to Dalston for a picnic', you go to Dalston for a picnic. Because your basement flat is cold and purple and smells of chip fat.

So I travelled far, far, far on the Tube to meet my friends for a picnic. We sat eating prawn cocktail crisps (possibly) and drinking warm white wine (probably) from plastic cups.

One of the earliest and best tips I received about my time in London was: take the bus. In any city, the bus gets you up and out of the tunnels. It allows you to see how the city streets roll out. It provides you with a three-dimensional map that teaches you that Charing Cross is actually only three minutes' walk from Embankment instead of a ten-minute sooty-sweat line-change.

After the picnic I approached a bus idling next to London Fields and asked if it was going to Tottenham Court Road.

'I'm heading back to the depot, love, but you can hop on for the ride if you like.'

I hesitated. I was shy in my early twenties. And a little nervous of kidnappers. But the warm white wine and a text from the blue-eyed one had emboldened me.

'All right then. Thank you.'

I made sure I sat halfway down the bus, to discourage both chat and kidnapping, and off we went. My own private double-decker charter through London. 'Not Taking Passengers' said the sign above the driver, as we whipped past bus stops and the Houses of Parliament. By the time we reached St Paul's I was grinning at passers-by. They stared at 'my' bus with its single passenger, a round happy face shining out the window, knowing already that this was a Moment I would not forget.

Lesson #48: Be aware of the Good Moments when you're in the midst of them.

Jim also took a bus to Tottenham Court Road. On day leave from hospital, he visited the dentist. It was foggy and his driver had to let him out before his stop:

I had read about London fogs, but always thought the descriptions exaggerated. Sure – thinks I to myself – it can't be any worse than a dark night. Now I take it all back … It was foggy when I went to see the dentist at Tottenham, but when I came out she'd thickened to what the Londoners call a 'black fog'.

I groped my way to the omnibus stand and found one of the celebrated London barouches bound down town. All the lights were lit, but ten feet away you could see nothing but a dull glow. Auto headlights looked like movies of themselves, taken at night.

The bus pushed cautiously along as far as Tottenham Court Rd, and there the lady in command decided she wouldn't go any farther. So I took the Tube, changed at Leicester Square, and finally arrived within about four blocks of 'home'.

Lesson #49: Travel with your eyes open.

My third London was up in the trees again, another small flat – this one in the leafy streets of Belsize Park. This was the flat where your blue-eyed father and I became Us and so of course I remember it being lighter, brighter and more full of love than the other bedrooms of the city.

Tom, the man from work with the blue, blue eyes, had moved into this flat the day we got (back) together. We'd (I'd) dillied, dallied and generally been a massive idiot for months, but we were finally locked and in love and the flat held us in a way we needed.

We lived beneath an extraordinarily noisy French family and would often wake to the sounds of young Thibault thrashing away at his xylophone at 6 am. Even in those new days of our relationship I'd gaze at Tom as he lay beside me half-asleep, and wonder if we'd have our own noisy toddler one day.

(Spoiler: you were quite noisy.)

It was a beautiful place to live, in this London that felt like home. We were close enough to Regent's Park Barracks that my walk to the Tube was sometimes accompanied by the hollow clop of horses heading up Haverstock Hill. The local square held pastel-painted shopfronts and our back window peeked into other people's Secret Gardens. The pub on the nearby Heath held a gap on the floor for an enormous wolfhound. No matter how busy the bar got, there was always empty airspace above the snoring beast. The flat looked out onto Belsize Square and a 150-year-old church that acted as our sedate timepiece as the months, then years, rolled on. Spring, summer, autumn, winter – I have photos of that same church in four different seasonal outfits. Richard Curtis had finally shown up.

The flat was halfway between the Northern and Jubilee lines and we'd walk uphill to one and downhill to the other. We didn't own a car and we didn't need to. Tubes, buses and – when we were feeling flush – a black cab. There were no Ubers back then, darling, can you imagine it?

The feeling of relief when an orange cab light floated into view on a dark and drizzling night is one I won't forget. In Australia, the taxis had seats pockmarked with cigarette burns and seatbelts that didn't work, and smelt of vomit tinged with Dettol. To this Australian, black cabs were like bouncy, rounded limousines. They still are.

As a young childless, carless couple, London was our walking city. Our calves were 20,000 steps-per-day tight and we didn't need to go to the gym after carrying three Budgens bags of groceries for kilometres. I became used to arriving home from anywhere with thigh muscles twitching and a faint sweat under whatever I was wearing. I believe now we call it 'incidental exercise'. Back then, it was 'leaving the flat'.

Lesson #50: Walk.

By then, in my fourth year in London, I was working in the old Carreras Cigarette Factory in Mornington Crescent, Camden.

It was a fantastically preserved Art Deco delight that included a pair of imposing two-and-a-half-metre-tall statues of black cats guarding the entrance. I could get from my front door to those cats in twenty-eight minutes of furious speed walking, which began by cresting Primrose Hill and finished by crossing the canal, surrounded by the blinding-white houses of Regent's Park.

Because I was too busy falling in love, making ads for Marks & Spencer and crafting my first ever iPod playlist, I neglected to realise I was walking the same streets your great-great-grandfather had, eighty-eight years earlier.

That hospital Jim had been sent to after being injured in Belgium was St Katherine's Lodge on Regent's Park. He stayed just over a month in London and as his shoulder repaired he spent his time sightseeing, theatre-going and party-hopping. Much like my time in the same city, but with more war:

> *Last night I sneaked out in a suit of civilian clothes and a bowler hat (borrowed from Bloomfield, the valet). Went to a low down dance at Kensington, where the ladies were all drunk. One of the aforesaid ladies declared her intention of staying with me, which I – being disgustingly sober – did not desire. I finally managed to lose her by stepping out of a train at a subway station, and arrived safe home, via the French window. And, Saturday night I went to a dawnce given by Lady Harcourt, – one of those feminine icebergs in a silk gown and a condescending atmosphere … Some sport, eh, what? I'm seeing all I can. Took in Westminster Abbey, London Bridge, and the Tower this week. Three or four more days will finish me here, and then – 'Quien Sabe?'*

I could tell you that *I* was never a lady drunk in a low-down dance, declaring intentions and wearing silk gowns. But I'd be lying to you and to my great-grampa. Or at least, I'd be lying about everything bar the silk gown.

Jim writes of feeding Regent's Park squirrels on the windowsills, catching the buses along Charing Cross Road and attending balls held at the hospital:

> *You know this 'lodge' was one of the hangouts of Charles I and he built the underground passage that leads from it to St. Katherine's Church. Since his time, the place has been enlarged and there is a ballroom that is a peach. So we got together, 'we' being the 'five patients' – those who can't get out of bed are known as 'dead 'uns' – and planned a shindig. Got the music from home talent in the three hospitals here. For partners we had the nurses and some few society ladies 'who take an interest in our poor, deah, wounded men.'*

The only reason I can forgive myself now that I didn't visit the property when I lived so close, is because it seems it was blown up in the next world war – by which time Jim was back in the US and his sons were fighting in his stead.

As a family of three, we have visited England, and London, many times since you were born. Each visit builds a different layer of understanding. You've covered your ears in the din of the Northern Line. You've bounced up high in the top-deck front-window seat of the bus (the gold-standard spot, where you fly rather than drive through the streets). You've breathed in the damp fog of Christmas air, where fairy lights finally make sense in the 4 pm twilight. You've experienced the magical season they call British summertime, lying in the grassy breeze where dragonflies and midges float on sunbeams.

There are so many corners of that city that I could hold your hand and point to. Some I have already. Many will have to wait until you're older. When I would say, had I the chance:

'There: there is where Mama learned to work, to love, to leave behind. Here: here is where I knew nothing. And left with everything.'

Letter Ten

Put your name on something

I hope, by now, these letters have begun to teach you something. I trust they've also shown you that this small group of ancestors are journeyers who like to stretch out into new climes. Yet we're also homebodies, people who relish the houses we have lived in and what they stand for. Who treasure the items inside, regardless of worth. Who notice the smallest lace trim, the gentlest brass glow and the softest soap scent.

It was in California in the mid-1950s, after four years working at his organisation's head office, when Buzz approached his boss and asked about the 'foreign service'. Namely because – as Virginia put it – he 'had something in mind and it wasn't a comfortable, suburban life'. Virginia expands on her husband's offer:

> *One night he came in from the office, mixed us a couple of martinis and asked,*
>
> *'How would you like to live in the shadow of a golden pagoda, have a nanny for the kids?'*
>
> *Well, who wouldn't! I didn't need the courage of my martini to help me answer, 'Yes!'*

Jim's manoeuvring paid off and in mid-February of 1958 he was offered a job in Melbourne, Australia. No pagodas to cast a shadow and probably no nanny, but an exciting adventure … we were delighted.

One of the reasons your family's stories tangle between Europe and the States and Australia, is the decision Buzz and Virginia took over that martini. They and their three children spent over a decade between three continents and six countries.

There is a quilt that I've run my hands over since I was born. It's Grama's – she embroidered it, stitching pictures of every house she's ever lived in. Black lace trim for iron lacework, knots for flowers on shrubs, the text of each address sewn in her own inimitable print. When you account for all the travelling she and Buzz did, it makes for a substantial undertaking. There are a dozen houses. Neatly embroidered hedges and windowpanes and chimneys. Australia, New Zealand, Kenya, Ghana, Sierra Leone, Connecticut.

The quilt now lies over Grama's bed in her nursing-home room, and is the main reason you're not allowed to play on her single bed without taking your shoes off.

You mightn't know this, given how few nursing homes you've visited, but Grama's is a lovely one. It does not smell of cabbage. The people who work there smile. You can't hear people moaning. There are copious plants around this nursing-home garden, and they are not plastic. When we visit we sit on her porch and have 'a little party'. Grama puts out a carved wooden bowl from Kenya, filled with potato chips. We have a glass of champagne, you have apple juice.

All of these things make it lovely, but not enough to graduate from the real world to her quilt. I might suggest, this is because her nursing-home room is a bedroom, but not a house. And certainly not a home.

The last home on the quilt is Shenzi, with all of its twenty-seven windows and sixteen doors. Shenzi, where my grandfather Jim became Buzz.

Buzz was so called because I named him that. The first grandchild always gets the privilege of naming the grandparent. Electric razor, lawnmower, an orchestra of tools in his shed: Buzz was always buzzing around their final home – Shenzi was a project never completed.

It wasn't until a decade after Buzz died that my stepfather, Ross, entered Shenzi for the first time. He spied an empty pipe sticking out of the wall, inside the open fireplace.

'Virginia, what's this?'

'Oh, it's a gas pipe. Buzz fed it into the mains so we could light the fire without using kindling.'

It was a live gas line. Piped into the open fireplace. Of the timber and grass matting house.

There was no regulator to prevent a flame going backwards. The only thing stopping the explosion was a dicey on/off valve. You, my darling – are lucky to be here for a number of reasons – including that the three generations above you weren't blown to kingdom come.

Yet that was the magic and mayhem of Shenzi. Buzz built into that original fibro house, out on top of it and all around it to suit himself, his wife, their children and grandchildren. It was a house constructed around the idiosyncrasies of a family. Virginia says of her husband:

> *Jim had built a lot of the house himself and it was a comfortable, loving old place because of this. If I wanted a shelf or cupboard in a convenient spot, Jim built me one. If we found a lead light window at a church fete, Jim could install it. He'd laid bricks, built decking round the pool, made me a greenhouse and a dove-cote, and now he was probably doing something more out in the workshop, where the children heard the sound of his electric drill.*

'Buzz!' they had to shout.

'Well, who are you?' he teased.

He was working on a better pulley for the tree house.

You can keep the Taj Mahal – Shenzi was filled with miniature shrines of love: some collected from around the world; most built in Buzz's workshop.

One day, Grama was sitting reading on the day bed that sat in the corner of the glassed-in front room of the house. She happened to mention that the windowsill wasn't deep enough to hold her cuppa. Buzz went out to his workshop and knocked up a little mug shelf. Just for Grama. To sit directly beside her elbow. Very small; only big enough to comfortably hold a coffee mug and nothing else. It stayed there until the house was no more.

Buzz's workshop was the most special place. It smelt of gasoline and fresh timber and Old Spice. There were black and white portrait 'studio' photos of impossibly beautiful women up high on the wall.

'Who are those ladies, Buzz?' I would ask.

'That's Audrey, we were engaged. And that's your grandmother. I married her.'

Grama would arrive around then, holding steaming cups of coffee. He'd wink at her and she'd wink at him and I was learning that the past was something to be welcomed, not hidden. And a good marriage seemed to be one that you could laugh at each other in.

Lesson #51: Never feel ashamed about your past. It's part of your present.

I was first introduced to a well-established family tradition at Shenzi. The masking tape. Small, torn pieces of yellowing adhesive stuck to the bottom of various objects around the house.

Blue biro printed carefully, the names of my mother, my aunt, my uncle. Some in Buzz's script, some in Grama's.

When Tom first visited Shenzi, I helped him across the threshold carefully, demonstrating how reverentially he should be treating this wonky old place. It wasn't too long before Grama asked him cheerfully, as he admired the souvenirs from the lives they'd led before, 'Do you like that? You can have it when I die!'

His British face twitched slightly, but given he'd already heard the line a few times from my mother, he wasn't shocked. It took him a few more years to actually put his name to anything, though.

Shenzi was demolished after Grama sold it in 2015. I'm pleased it's gone; pleased I don't have to imagine another family sowing their own memories over our established ones. The plot is only 600 metres from Mum and Ross's house in the same town, but I haven't visited it. I don't need to see a modern monolith sitting atop Buzz's shed, Grama's greenhouse and the swimming pool-shaped hole that Grama turned into a veggie patch after Buzz died.

Grama left Shenzi when she was eighty-eight. I believe it was one of her greatest gifts to her family: to manage her own departure. She walked into her nursing home before she needed it. No-one else had to make the decision on her behalf and, while not a material object, that was one of the greatest gifts of all.

Lesson #52: Leave before you have to.

After Grama left Shenzi, we visited the empty house for one last time. As you toddled through the echoing rooms, I took photos of every small thing I could see. Footworn steps, 1970s-psychedelic curtains, stained-glass windows, Buzz's shed door. The things that people don't photograph are often the corners they miss the most.

I am telling you all about Shenzi and what it meant to me and our family, because it's gone. There is another home that is still standing, not too far from us now. And, as I write, it is still occupied by our folk. Number 38 was my home from when Mum and Dad moved in, in 1983, to when I left in 2003. When Mum leaves it, I will need a photo album of one hundred pages to hold a record of every small piece of that house that is so special to me. I will click the shutter desperately and still miss almost everything. That house is the anchor to my life. It is so much closer to my heart and Kate's and yours and all of the family. So close, that I can't really bear to look directly at it.

Lesson #53: Leave before you have to.
But it's okay to never let go.

Like many elderly people who fold up their lives and pack them into a single room, Grama had to give away much of her history. Now she lives in a room set along a hallway of pastels and beeping. Her ninety-four years are marked by a filing cabinet with important family documents (including the original copies of the letters her father wrote from the Front). There is a minibar, always stocked with a bottle of champagne. Four glass flutes. An en suite with wall-mounted hospital soap. A shelf of photographs.

Her father wrote to her mother, long before she was born:

> *Your picture hangs now in my billet, a little, stone floored room on the Rue de la Fontaine of a French village. Besides that your picture floats before car windows and dances on the waves and smiles from dark roadsides when troops march by. At least, it does all these things for me, always.*

If you had to curate a lifetime of objects to fit into one single room, what would it contain? Of the thousand books in our house, which ten would make the cut? Which paintings would be given the precious wall space? Is there one rug, one rug you would want to walk on for the rest of your days?

I don't know what would make it into my room, my dear. But I have a roll of masking tape and a biro, and together you and I are going to walk through some houses and claim some tokens of life and love.

I would like to start with a mauve glass bottle.

When Virginia was little, she was as enamoured by her parents' belongings as any child is:

> *The house held possessions with which I was fascinated. I'd caress the assorted mauve glass bottles on Mother's dressing table as I watched her set her hair. The stipulated waves of fashion were disciplined by a viscous fluid she made herself by boiling thin pieces of some sort of tree bark sold for that purpose … Daddy's treasures were even more intriguing. Like an incredible leaf he'd acquired in France during the war. A loving message was written in French on the centre, the rest had been somehow rotted so only a delicate filigree of veins remained in leaf shape. Also from France was a music box topped with a large, square tile depicting [the fortified gates of the town] La Ferté-Bernard.*

I've held this music box, as have you. It's heavy.

This box is one of the objects that has made it to Grama's nursing-home room. When we visit, she lifts it slowly, ceremoniously, onto her bed and we lean in to see its beautiful inlaid porcelain painting and carefully polished timber. It has heft, and bulk, and I wonder just how Jim managed to get it all the way back from France in 1919 without it breaking. When Jim talked of the souvenirs he had, and lost, the fact that the music box remains is most impressive. Mostly because of its size, but also because his hospital stay in 1918 lightened his load a little.

> *'It's taking some time to get [your] letters, but I've lost everything I had – even your address. It's a good thing I had a money belt on me with 1500 Francs in it. I guess the hospital orderlies*

overlooked that when I was unconscious. They took everything else … including some souvenirs. So when I come home, I won't bring you any souvenirs – except a bigger love than ever.'

We have our mauve glass bottle, and a music box. Shall we add the nude lady?

Her name is *Simone*, and she's a sculpture by Australian artist Peter Corlett. Mum purchased her in the 1990s and she's stood in Mum's living room ever since. She is life-size and lifelike. Completely nude, except for a pair of small heels. Her arms are uplifted; her hands hold her hair. Her hips jut, her eyes look directly ahead, she has a scar on her pelvis. None of us blink at Simone, and she never blinks back. We are confused when visitors are confused. Even you, now, with young friends who giggle and blush at the naked woman in your grandmother's house. 'That's Simone,' you say matter-of-factly. 'She's always been here.'

I was aware of Corlett's work from a young age, as most children in Victoria would have been, because he cast the many nudes that graced the original Children's Museum in Melbourne. Men and women. In wheelchairs and not. Young, old, drooping, dimpled, hairy, smooth and sagging. Completely naked, completely lifelike people. I look back now and see a rather white-bread group, but it can't be overstated just how formative an experience it was to see the nude form in all shapes – destigmatised and normalised.

Lesson #54: Treat your house like a museum and your objects like artefacts. Regardless of their value.

We have added a sculpture of a naked woman to our bottle and music box. I would like to include a brocade ball gown. Virginia wore it to the 1961 Fourth of July Ball in Wellington, New Zealand. It may be a touch scuffed at the hem, but given her entrance, this is the charm. Because she arrived at the ball via a fire escape, through a window into the men's toilets and down the lift. Also, to reference a twenty-first century meme: 'It has pockets!'

> *After work Buzz would often go with his friends for a drink at the Grand Hotel [in Wellington]. He'd park his car in the lot off the street which ran behind the hotel, level with the second floor. By climbing up the fire escape and crawling through the window of the men's room on that floor he gained access to the hotel without going all the way around to the front door on the lower street. He'd take the lift down to the bar and meet his friends.*
>
> *The Fourth of July Ball was held in the Grand Hotel and Buzz parked, as usual, in the back parking lot. I was in my ivory brocade ball gown and beaver coat with pockets stuffed with the wine for the evening. (Going into a pub carrying wine seems odd now, but that was required or permitted in those days.) Up the fire escape we went then through the window into the second floor men's toilet and down the lift to an elegant ball.*

Lesson #55: The right accessories ensure a fabulous entrance.

A nude sculpture with an ivory ball gown draped beside it. A mauve glass bottle sitting next to a music box. Can you see the masking tape? They all have your name on them today. Now I would like to add an orchid. And because we are playing pretend, we can imagine the flower as white and velvety as it was the day that Jim gifted it to his Kay, on a wedding anniversary during the war. The *second* war, the one to which Jim will have sent his sons with his own battles fresh in his mind. We have Grama to thank for an account of this gift-giving ceremony:

> *Daddy had taken Mother to dinner at the Fairmont and presented her with a corsage from Podesta Baldocchi, the best florist in the city. Nestled in the box beside the white orchid was the deed to the block of land in Palo Alto they had always wanted. Though*

> *construction couldn't start until materials became available, the fun of planning carried them through the dark days of their mothers' deaths and worry about [their son] Carter flying over Japan.*

Jim had marched his way through blood and mud and rain and fear. But he still carried a music box home from war. He hoped there would be a woman waiting for him, to turn the key and listen to the song.

His sons were deployed in their own war, but he still bought the deed for a family home. He hoped his children would all eventually return to his wife and himself, under that one roof.

This is the power that being optimistic and brave can give you. It's the power of hope. Of course, Jim and Kay could not live *in* the property deed that lay beside the orchid, but their future did. And that is what a home can be – and what a home should be. It does not have to be everything, straightaway. It just needs to be a place where the future *might* happen. Walls and a roof that may grow to contain love, and family, and joy, and French music boxes.

It is okay to have a shitty first car, or first love, or first house. You just need to leave space for the hope to sit.

Lesson #56: Hope is strength.

When Tom and I first lived together, we served all our drinks in one set of glasses. When I was washing up in the kitchen that doubled as a dining, living and laundry, I daydreamed of being grown-up enough to have glasses not only for water, but for wine too. When we moved into the first house we owned together, the small wall-mounted heaters only managed to warm up the twenty square centimetres directly around the grate. We woke up on our first morning in that single-fronted cottage on Earl Street with our breath fogging. Inside. Buzz's first home with Grama wasn't too different:

> *[Virginia and I] were married in 1950 at her folks' house. We rented a one bedroom house in the middle of an apricot orchard in San Jose. The bathroom was so small you could sit on the toilet, brush your teeth and take a shower at the same time.*

Life is infinitely more fun if you've had to wade through some rubbish to get to the good bits. I'm not suggesting penitence, just … don't expect to hit all of your highs early on. As Buzz's gravestone says, 'Life is a matter of contrast'.

Lesson #57: Leave yourself somewhere to go.

A nude sculpture, an ivory ball gown, a mauve glass bottle, and a music box that holds a white orchid and the deed to a block of land. Hold them safe, bring them close – understand what they are and what they aren't.

Buzz once played a similar game to the one we are playing now, in New Zealand in the 1960s:

> *We found a wonderful old place to rent. It was big and had been lived in by a woman who was given the house completely furnished when she married as a young girl. She lived there until she was eighty five and had to go into a nursing home. We moved in the day she moved out and everything but clothing was there. For entertainment we'd open a drawer or two on the weekend and examine all the items. It was fascinating.*

'You can have it when I die' is a familiar refrain in our family. It may sound morbid, but it means 'Let me live on'; 'Thank you for appreciating this object'; 'Thank you for recognising who I was before I was Mother/Grama/Nursing Home Resident'.

Because that is what objects are, my love. They are representations of who we were when we acquired them. Who we wanted to be, when we took them home. Who we loved, when we received them. I do not subscribe to this 'material things don't matter' nonsense. Material things *do* matter when they're bound to the people we love and the feelings we had and the memories we made.

Lesson #58: Don't be afraid of of sentimentality – allow your memories to take physical form.

Letter Eleven

Your heart will break

This is the letter to read when you've had your heart obliterated. But this is *not* a letter about love or lovers. Heartbreak can too often be kidnapped by the heartbreaker, which is to say, a person who has cheated you, or left you, or just been cruel.

No. Allow heartbreak to be about *you* and *your* heart. That is the shortest path to the restoration of that special organ (and even better, the growth of it). Because the times when I've been truly heartbroken have not been limited to a lovers' break-up or a romantic rejection. It has been bigger than that. Heartbreak is about when life has not continued on the path we were expecting. It is a despair of loss, a swallow of betrayal and a rage at a life that is not going to plan.

I have experienced many small moments of heartbreak in my life. You will too. All of us have, this bunch of family who've made it through – all of us have broken in more ways than we can remember, and in more ways than we have told each other.

We weren't okay. We were okay. It will be the same for you.

Lesson #59: You will break.

We build muscle by exercising, by shredding microtears in our tissue. As these tiny rips in our bodies heal, they build muscle – stronger, tougher, thicker. A heart is just the same. A heart that is crisscrossed with the scar tissue of heartbreak is a heart that has been expanded with love and joy.

Lesson #60: You will break, but don't be afraid.

There have been four types of heartbreak that I've been scarred by. This doesn't mean you will be injured in the same way, by the same thing. That's the wonderful thing about our hearts – they are ours, and what happens to them is as unique as knots in the scars left behind. So I share this letter not as a warning of what to avoid, but as a demonstration of pain that did not mean the end. Not the end for me, or anyone else along our family line, who had – or still have – scars beating in their chest.

The barbed heartbreak of betrayal.

In 2002, I was sitting in the front seat of my mate's vintage Fiat. It smelt of petrol and leather and cigarettes and all the other things I imagined vehicles from the 1970s smelt like. The wipers squealed the rain away. I felt the citrus prickle of adrenaline under my arms, and sour saliva filling my mouth. I was going to be sick.

'I'm so sorry,' she said.

'No, I'm glad I'm hearing it from you.'

And I was. Having one of my dearest and bests telling me that my boyfriend at the time had been shagging everyone else was the only way I wanted to find out that gross, sad news. But even before she could tell me anything more, before *he* would tell me anything more, I was already scrabbling at ways to make it all go away.

That night, the rain came down and my stomach dropped with it. I couldn't bear to lose the relationship. Instead, I forgave him. I heaped my forgiveness onto his betrayal. But even then, deep down, I knew he didn't deserve me feeling that I would do 'anything, *anything*' to have him back. To have it The Way It Was. I just didn't understand then how much there was to forgive.

Lesson #61: 'The Way It Was' is rarely 'The Way It Should Be'.

Later, as I sat in my own car after a thorough and necessary STD check, I wished I could rescind my forgiveness. And almost immediately, I realised I could.

Lesson #62: No-one can take your forgiveness without your consent.

My mother has coped with more than her fair share of heartbreak. But what is a 'fair share' of heartbreak? Two betrayals? Twenty losses? Do we have an allocated number at birth? All I know is I have seen her shift herself through heartbreak a number of times. Certainly enough to have a dedicated fan club among the scandalmongers of our proverbial village.

One of the things I love the most about my mother is her resolute stubbornness in refusing bitterness. To remain open to love, wonder and joy – even after being on the receiving end of 'more than her fair share'. I like to think it's because she understands she is worthy of the right kind of love. And chose to keep seeking it.

That, and because she had children to keep turning up for. As on the day that Dad left, when she sat shell-shocked at our kitchen table, being comforted by an old friend:

> *'When my husband left I had the first decent night's rest in twenty years.' [My friend] grins like a fiend, 'You won't know yourself, love.'*

> *I've had to be so many different people, I don't know myself now. Who will it be next? I breathe out … and in again. It's getting easier. Then I remember Ella and Jim. I have to tell Ella and Jim.*

And there began a specific heartbreak for Mum. She had two kids and a decade of marriage to heal around.

My early heartbreak was soured by infidelity and the realisation I had wasted some of the best years my boobs would ever have. However, it was a break that repaired itself much more quickly than I expected. Looking back, it's not surprising.

Lesson #63: Your heartbreak will last exactly as long as it's meant to.

Not long after the night of the Fiat and the rain and the forgiveness, I also asked myself, 'Who will I be next?' Because I had been in a relationship since I was just-eighteen, that question was extraordinarily thrilling. I was twenty-one and falling in love with *myself* for the first time. I didn't know who I would be next, I just knew I would like her. New clothes, new hair … that didn't matter. I was wearing new skin! I felt beautiful, I felt unfamiliar, I felt like the Next Who I was becoming. I remember the lyrics of more songs, the taste of more food, the smell of more nights from that time than I do from the preceding years. It's because I was waking up. And it was the most wonderful feeling.

Lesson #64: The After is often so much better than the Before.

When Jim was in France, he and Kay seem to have had that conversation every pair of long-distance lovers has, eventually. I can't be sure of Kay's question, but Jim's response doesn't leave much in doubt:

Would it be strange – as the world sees things – if you were to let the thought of me slip some of these times? Not at all. And I am thousands of miles from home, an officer of a victorious army in a celebrating land where the eternal feminine is hell and the straight and narrow is as rare as sauerkraut at a French dinner.

Oh Jim. If this is an appeasement I'd hate to see a confession. But hold on, he continues:

Yet I'm straight – as far as the Greater Sins are concerned – and even if I were not – or even if you were not – we'd still swing back together and hit the same trail. My imagination fails to show me any situation which would change the desire I now have to hold you tight in my arms and bury my face in your hair – whether you'd had a shampoo or not.

There's my platform. Do you vote with me, Prairie Lady?

They did swing back together, and remained married for nearly seven decades. Yes, my love – she voted with him. And god, wouldn't we all?

*

I don't hold a scar from my first heartbreak. If I ever did, it's long faded away. The scar from my parents' heartbreak beats in my chest instead. My father turned seventy this year. In his speech, he thanked the two mothers of his five children, women who were both absent from the table. He did this despite the fact he had gone on to marry and love someone else. It was an acknowledgement that was unexpected and unasked, which made it all the more powerful. On that evening, that particular heart-scar faded a little more.

Lesson #65: It is never too late.

The dulled heartbreak of homesickness.

July 2003. I had been in London for a month. My boyfriend left for work every morning, and I tried very hard to do the things that I knew would tether me to the day. I washed. I put on lipstick. I left that small Top Floor Flat. I made the single coffee I could afford last as long as I could without the barista frowning at me. The cafe was on the corner of Parkway and Arlington Road, and even though it was high summer I sat inside because I was still confused about whether I was in a safe area or not. This is what being a foreigner is. You don't know the rules of where you live, and where you fit in. I sipped my coffee. I listened to traffic. I wrote a list:

> ***Things I wish I could buy***
> *Hairspray*
> *A magazine*
> *Six beers for my boyfriend*
> *Flowers for the flat*
> *Food and drink for the flat*
> *'Lady Sings the Blues' CD*

I had never had less money. In emigrating, I watched my savings go from Australian dollars to English pounds: in the flick of a finger, paper to ash. I could still afford rent and bills and food, but only with the help of my boyfriend. It stung to be dependent, and it made the homesickness so much worse.

In hindsight, turning up in a new city without a job or a friend or somewhere to go during the day was a challenging decision. Unsurprisingly, that's when the homesickness began.

Homesickness can be the process of seeking out environments that you hope tells strangers what kind of person you are. Being without a fixed and obvious identity forced me to cultivate a more outward-facing personality. Eye contact, smiles, small talk: I pushed out signals like an animal pulsing out pheromones.

'Be my friend! Like me! Know who I am!'

That first year, the homesickness was as bright and sharp as a needle. It was an acute pain, but it was also the easiest to resolve. As soon as I found a job, I stopped sitting in corner cafes writing lists. I dunked myself deep into the city and its people, avoiding the Aus-ghettos of Clapham and Shepherd's Bush. I'd go for long stretches without talking to another Aussie. It suited me – most of my countrymen were quick to complain about the weather, the expense, the terrible coffee … it felt like a vortex back to those tough early days straight off the plane. I had also realised something simple: if I avoided all places and people that reminded me of home, then I couldn't be homesick!

Lesson #66: Sometimes, denial is necessary.

Buzz, Virginia, Mum and her brother arrived in Australia in the late autumn of 1958 'with only their sunburns to keep them warm'. You can't imagine a more faraway place than grey, winter-logged Melbourne compared to the sunny skies of California. It was their first overseas posting after deciding to do away with the 'comfortable, suburban life' they had been cultivating.

After three weeks at the Chevron Hotel on St Kilda Road, the family of four rented a Toorak maisonette. Grama remembers:

> *It was cold, very cold. Every night we'd pile every coat and sweater we had with us on top of the beds and still we were shivering. The walls seeped cold into the unheated rooms. Even the decor was cold.*

Things felt hard for the young family. The couple established Buzz's 'Frozen Juice Syndrome' and its cure. If only I'd known about it in my first year overseas.

> *[In Melbourne] some things were unobtainable, items we'd been used to such as frozen orange juice, instant coffee, soft toilet paper and cake mixes. But Buzz wisely set forth an edict which combated the 'frozen orange juice syndrome'. We were never to complain about the cold or lack of some American foodstuff. Speaking of it, even within the family, gave the problem importance which might lead to dissatisfaction with our situation. We looked around us, saw Australians living very well indeed on what was available. We later saw Americans in various parts of the world suffering from the frozen orange juice syndrome so severely they eventually had to be sent home.*

The next, deeper stage of longing is harder to kick. It is a dull ache. And one I don't think ever truly disappeared during my time away. It certainly ebbed, flowed, and eventually rolled in tides that I learned to swim through. Yet my diaries and letters and all my writing from those four years have a constant drizzle of homesickness through them.

I travelled back to Australia for good in 2007, without Tom. The homesick heartbreak had become too much, and I had become monochrome and muted. I returned expecting the shining skies of Melbourne, where I'd last lived as an in-love child-adult who didn't know much about the world. And it was not the same. It was four years later. In the dipped-mattress, beside the pink oleander and the twist of a tram squeal outside, I found it wasn't my room anymore. I wrote another list:

> ***Things I need to do***
> *Sit-ups, lunges*
> *Less than an hour of computer a day*
> *Don't overeat*
> *Moisturise*
> *Write one thing every day*

Lesson #67: If you ever feel homesick, consider what are you actually sick for.

Jim's parents left Maryland in 1902 for those shining skies of California. And they were homesick. Homesick for the lovely green summertime woods filled with family and picnics. So sick that they packed up all they had moved to San Jose and returned home to Maryland after eight years away. But, oh no:

> *[Four years later] they found that a strange thing had happened. In spite of all their homesickness, and their distress at not having their families and relatives around them, or the lovely leafy woods in the summertime to have picnics in, and all that sort of talk – in spite of all that, they had become Californians. So, in the summer of 1914, they left Maryland and came back to California.*

Homesickness is a terrible beast, because it makes you sick not for the home you left behind, but the one you're slowly realising you can never return to.

Homesickness can also be an ablution. It can be a hurt that propels you to seek something better – to move forward rather than go back. It is a scar in your heart that you can feel with a smile; that reminds you where you once were, and who you have become. What did Jim say to Kay, all those years ago?

> *No, dear girl, you don't seem dream like, nor far away to me. I know you're there, waiting for me. If it weren't for you – America and home would mean nothing to me. I never was homesick for home. Now I am homesick for you.*

The empty heartbreak of longing.

The feeling of not being able to have a child, when you want to have a child, is horrible. It creates such sadness. I hope you never experience this. But if you do, know that I understand, and that I am sorry.

Primary infertility was one of the most spiritually painful things I've experienced. Even before your father and I were married we started to try for a baby. I was twenty-seven. Nothing happened. I thought, in all those years that we had studiously ignored proper birth-control methods, that we were just 'really lucky'. Turns out, we were just 'really infertile'.

Those 'trying' years were filled with a longing I wouldn't wish on anyone. Infertility is almost worse than cancer (and I can say that). With most cancers, you get kick-in-the-guts news every few months, or less. With infertility, you get kicked Every. Single. Month. For years. Because living with infertility is living with a white noise of grief and desperate wanting. It is a cycle of hope and failure, where you wind your own roller-coaster up so high, that every month your entire future climbs and crumbles before you. And this particular shitty roller-coaster is ridden *in public*, surrounded by people getting the exact thing you're wanting. Every swollen belly, online announcement, baby shower, is tainted with the sour tang of defeat.

Lesson #68: Never ask, 'When are you having kids?' You have no idea where they have been, or where their hearts are.

Much like my cancer diagnosis, I chased down our fertility difficulties with a fervour some might mistake for desire.

'It's like you actually *want* something to be wrong with you!' laughed a colleague, after I booked in with my gyno after only (only?) a year of trying and failing.

(I suspect this person ended up in the pandemic camp of, 'If we stop testing right now, we'd have very few cases …' but I digress.)

I very much did not want something to be wrong with me. Instead, I wanted a baby. We both did. We wanted to link ourselves together with a human that we had helped bring into the world. That want is so primal.

There were countless days when I would steady myself in the public eye of work, the tram, the walk home – only to fall through the door, letting go with Tom once I was private. I'd weep over whichever form my 'failure' had taken: a negative urine test, the gentle, 'I'm sorry' call from the fertility nurse, or just the innocuous arrival of yet another period. I would howl my day into a pillow while Tom stroked my back.

This city still holds pockets of heartbreak-memories for me. A curve of road, a traffic light. One intersection by the Yarra River still shoots me back to a particular afternoon, wailing at the steering wheel as I left behind another negative pregnancy test. Oh, that pain. The pain of wanting something so very badly. I remember every aching minute.

My girl, I have never wanted anything so much as we wanted you.

IVF is an expensive, precise game of psychological torture. You grit your teeth and plough through the bureaucracy of medicine. Your life is dictated by calendars and notebooks and sums of money that take your breath away. We had the misery and privilege of undertaking IVF for a long time. We stopped, we rested, we started again. And somewhere in the mess of all of that, I became pregnant, naturally. We did nothing special to make this happen. It was, as a doctor told me later, a complete medical anomaly.

Lesson #69: You are, scientifically and objectively speaking, a miracle.

Falling pregnant completely unexpectedly was wonderful. Although I did spend the whole pregnancy terrified that you'd fall out as surprisingly as you fell in. That's why I still recall when I first felt you flutter, deep in my belly. I was travelling on the number 16 tram as it rolled over the Princes Bridge. It was early morning and the upside-down brown of the Yarra was twinkling under the rowers, when I realised the feathery movements weren't my body, but yours. This was the first time I understood you were your own self – a realisation that typifies the journey of motherhood. It is a rolling dichotomy of ownership and loss. It is saying a thousand minuscule goodbyes, all the while knotting silk threads of connection between the two of you. The irony is not lost on me that you're reading this and I've gone and died. That's what this book is, in case you hadn't realised. Twenty-seven knotted silk threads.

Secondary infertility is a different type of heartbreak, rather like carrying around a little growl of sadness. Small, but there, nevertheless. So although we had you, our miracle child, we continued to thump along with IVF.

*

While no-one ever said it, I did wonder if after having one surprise baby it was a teensy bit selfish to try and roll a miracle again. And this time around, there was a louder expectation from some around us that we should 'just relax and it'll happen again'.

Lesson #70: If you're managing infertility and someone tells you to 'just relax and it'll happen', you have your mother's permission to scream. Loudly.

Cancer kicked us off our next IVF train. The requirement for me to start radiation and chemo as soon as possible made that decision – swiftly and deftly – on our behalf. At the time I marvelled at how clean it felt to hear, 'You will not have any more children.' I went from wearing the nametag of 'unexplained infertility' to 'premature menopause' in one week. Yes, there was that growly sadness. But also ... there was relief.

I know it's a cop-out, but it was a comfort to hand the future of my (in)fertility to someone else. Being freed from the decision-making around IVF was incredibly liberating. Someone else made the call for us, and we were allowed to sink into the life I think we'd subconsciously already decided to be happy with.

There was no more wondering, no more supplements, no more calendars. And no more heartbreak.

Three years later and we are permanently a single-child family – something I don't need to tell you. We are a family of three piles of washing on the kitchen table and three fields in online booking forms. That particular heartbreak has gone, but the scar remains. It aches, like joints before rain, when I see a baby photo of you, or hear you talk of your own single-child loneliness.

Sometimes, at that last point, I understand with a heaviness that this heartbreak seems to have been passed onto you. You and I are tethered by this particular silk thread, one scar tied to another. I'm so sorry I couldn't give you a sibling, my darling. I'm sorry you feel the pain of wanting. Hopefully one day your heartbreak will become just a heartbeat in a heart-scar, like mine is. Hopefully.

The breathless heartbreak of loss.

Loss that comes as a shock hits you sharply in the sternum.

It makes this sound: 'Oof'.

That is the sound of your body processing the news before your brain has.

When someone dies suddenly, parts of your body will separate. Your stomach and your heart and your brain and your limbs will all be floating, adrift, torn apart by shock. All parts of you will process the news in different ways and along different timelines.

Lesson #71: Shock will tear you apart. You will come back together. Differently, but together.

Loss that is expected doesn't hurt any less. It just hurts differently. Loss that is expected places itself on your shoulder like an icy hand.

It makes this sound: 'Oh'.

That is the sound of receiving a grief that you knew was coming, and that you thought you were ready for. It is the sound of realising you could never be ready for it.

Lesson #72: Being prepared will not protect you.

> *This stupid French driver got lost and went through the same town twice. The poor captain in the lower stretcher kept choking on blood; I tried to reach down with my good left hand and hold his head up so that he could breathe. When we arrived, I made the usual statement of, 'Oh, take care of this poor fellow first, as he needs it more than I do.'*
>
> *The orderlies looked at him and said, 'He's been dead for an hour.'*

I haven't been in the midst of death, holding up its head, like Jim did during his time at war. I have not sat at the bedside of a dying husband and father, like Virginia and Kate did, with Buzz. I cannot tell you how your heart will scar after I am gone.

But I have seen and smelt the grief that death will bring. I have held the heartbreak that death leaves behind. I own the scars that heartbreak brought. The one thing I can tell you, is that as sure as there is death, and grief; there is life, and – stay with me here – laughter.

Lesson #73: A sense of humour will help light your way.

The way someone dies can leave behind different volumes of grief. There is a great power in acceptance, which is not to be confused with surrender. Understanding your place in the process of death can help those around you. *Laughing* at this place, can help you even more.

You come from stock that can laugh through heartbreak. That is our gift to you. Take it.

Buzz explained:

> *Virginia gave me a [burial] plot on my 60th birthday. I went down to the cemetery trust … to pick [one] out.*
>
> *The young lady said, 'Here's the chart.'*
>
> *It was in bad shape, it was parchment and you couldn't read it. It was badly marked up, pieces of paper stuck to it with sticky tape and arrows.*
>
> *I said, 'I can't pick a plot from this chart,' and she said, 'No-one can, we'll see you up there in fifteen minutes.'*
>
> *I found a spot on top of the hill. You could see the Rip and you could see the Bay.*
>
> *I said, 'This is where I want to be.'*

It's a beautiful spot. We visit Buzz often, picking our way through the graves. We took a photo of you next to his grey headstone when you were little, asleep in your pusher. Buzz had an excellently morbid sense of humour and he would have liked that even after death, he was still making new entries in the family photo album.

> *I picked a plot and she gave me a receipt for $54.00, imagine that.*
>
> *I said, 'Hey, I think I'll take twenty plots and build a house on it.'*
>
> *She said, 'I don't think you can do that.'*
>
> *I said, 'Well maybe I'll take three or four and build a sort of mausoleum with a couple of TV screens and people can put twenty cents in it and watch videos of me and my life story.'*

> *I am not sure the young lady appreciated my sense of humour. I picked a plot and on the bottom of the receipt she wrote Methodist.*
>
> *I said, 'I'm not a Methodist, I'm an Agnostic,' and she said, 'Well, you're a Methodist now because you're in the Methodist section.'*

Buzz does not have a mausoleum, but he has a family, and we put twenty cents into each other and tell stories often.

This is very deliberately a letter for you about heartbreak and what it can feel like, rather than how you can rid yourself of it. Because you can't. All you can do is run your fingers along the small roped scars and say, 'Ah. So this is what it feels like.'

Letter Twelve

Some little things that take too long to learn

Tweezers.

Tweezers are where this entire book began. Not long after I was diagnosed, I began my daily radiation treatments. At my request, the medical team sat down and helped me schedule the appointments around school pick-up. You were one term into your Prep year, and I wanted to make sure that despite cancer treatment, I was in the playground for as many afternoons as possible. It also gave me something to do besides Googling my new life expectancy and sweeping the floors.

As the weeks wore on and the radiation made me more tired, I would get home from hospital, set my alarm for 2.45 pm, and settle in for a nap.

Lesson #74: If you are setting your alarm for a time after midday it may be the sign of depression, old age or that you're smoking too much weed. Whichever it is, it's best to check in on yourself.

I'd set my alarm for 2.45 pm, wake up, put some make-up on (so other mothers wouldn't stop me in the playground and weep), and drive the five minutes to pick up my little Preppie. Walking any distance was difficult at this stage.

It was during that short drive one day that I spied a few of my stray eyebrow hairs in the rearview mirror. Because there is a special way that the light hits your face in a car that doesn't seem to be replicated anywhere else. Some kind of sorcery occurs when you combine visor mirrors and sunlight that means, no matter how hard you try, you'll never see your face like you do in the car. So whether it's eyebrow hairs, chin hairs (you're welcome) or just a stray poppyseed in a tooth – it's always the car where you need an implement on hand to take advantage of said lighting, and enact any emergency tweaks.

'Bugger.'

No tweezers.

Then, from that moment to the next I fell to thinking about dying early, dying soon, and not being able to tell you all the things that you need to know.

Lesson #75: Keep tweezers in your car.

Dizzying leaps of logic happen often when you're thirty-six, irradiated and full of fear. I had a little cry as I drove towards school, but by then I was into my third week of treatment so I'd already switched to waterproof mascara.

Standing in the playground on the four-square markings in the brutal autumn wind, one of the mothers approached. Seeing my (made-up) face she exclaimed, 'But you're looking so *well*!'

She clearly couldn't see my eyebrows.

*

Sweet girl. If you thought this collection was going to be all Meaningful Lessons and Worthy Teachings, consider this the rug-pull letter. Because there are some crucial lessons I must pass on that don't involve life, death or any of the big cymbal-crash moments in between.

These lessons may seem flippant, but some of them may be the most important I give you. They include but aren't limited to tweezers, cotton knickers and the significance of good lighting. How not to be a snob – but also, the importance of linen napkins and having fresh flowers in the house whenever you can afford it. And, I will tell you to write thank you letters.

Lesson #76: Write thank you letters. For gifts, for hospitality, for just being a friend.

It was my twenty-first birthday party, in the back yard at number 38, and my father and future stepfather were downstairs, squaring off like two bulls over the hors d'oeuvres. I was upstairs, bent over my bed in my room. Three women (including my mother) sipped champagne while a friendly GP stuck my bottom with a needle filled with antibiotics. I'd come down with such a severe case of cystitis in the afternoon that by 8 pm I could barely stand, never mind circulate through the plastic marquee. The drugs kicked in and I managed to get back downstairs to finish the rest of my birthday party in all its mid-August chill and glory. There were a number of lessons learned that evening, but the most immediately useful was the one whispered to me by another party guest over a flute of bubbly:

Lesson #77: Wee. Straight after sex.

It's not glam, but boy – those are four words I wish someone had said to me much sooner than they did. I was twenty-one and I had been told the trick to avoiding 80 per cent of the UTIs I had been grappling with ever since I'd started having sex.

So I'm saying it to you. Even if it makes you feel a bit squeamish, hearing it from your mother. If you're having penis–vagina intercourse then go for a wee as soon as you can afterwards.

And drink plenty of water. You'll avoid a lot of pain. Literally.

While we're on the subject of fannies, thrush is another treat those of us blessed with a vagina can get dumped with. I certainly did, particularly during IVF and, later, chemotherapy treatments.

Lesson #78: Stick with cotton knickers.

If your undies are making your bits sweaty, you're on a one-way path to Canesten Land. Best keep things breathing. Also:

Lesson #79: Popping a good probiotic on the reg is good for your whole body, not just your bits.

Now, from one type of cotton to another – let's discuss napery.

Lesson #80: Set the table with cloth napkins.

Linen, if you can afford it. But cotton, muslin; it doesn't matter. No whites – you're not a masochist. Any meal served with a proper napkin tastes 11 per cent better, which isn't much unless, like me, you are a substandard cook and need all the help you can get. Mum has always had cloth napkins in a beautiful print similar to Grama's, of browns, reds and oranges. Will you remember mine? A rainbow of colours and patterns. Cheerful, and excellent at hiding sauce stains.

I have some of Grama's linen placemats – stiff with starch and almost transparent with age. They are monogrammed with 'EDE', which we think references the initials of Buzz's adopted mother. They're kept in the back of the laundry cupboard and to my great shame I've never used them. Until today: right now I'm going to pull them out and you, your father and I will eat dinner on them this evening. It is Monday. We're having tacos. It is not a special occasion and that is okay.

Lesson #81: Don't save things for 'best'.

Soaps, shoes, earrings, words. It's ironic that often the most special and revered items that we own are the ones we leave in cabinets and cupboards. Wear the sparkly shoes, dangle the heavy earrings from your lobes, shout out, 'You're my best!' as if it's your very last chance to. I have come across so many different 'bests' that I've never used. Some I've grown out of. Some have grown out of me. It's a tragedy to realise nothing was 'best' enough until it was too late.

Lesson #82: Only gamble what you're willing to lose.

I don't just mean that in the literal sense, I've never had a problem with gambling myself. Your great-great-grandfather learned his lesson the hard way. He was eighteen and completing a stint in the National Guard:

> *Here it was midnight, and I had lost all my money. I had even hazarded my saddle, in my last gambling instinct, and I had lost that. So I hiked four miles across the desert, after midnight, where I knew there was an artillery outfit. I was able to steal a saddle, and carry it back. And every step I took, it got heavier and heavier, but I was ready at 7.30 for parade. I had my saddle. But every step I took, I swore to myself, 'I'm gonna quit gambling; it's not what it's cracked up to be.' So that was a good lesson, in that I've never gambled since.*

No. What I mean is: don't play a hand you don't have.

Don't threaten to resign in order to get a pay rise. Don't break up with a lover in order to have them fall in love with you. Don't slam a door in the expectation someone will come after you.

I met your father when I was very young. I hadn't yet quite grasped that every fight wasn't the end to every relationship. One evening we went to bed in a quarrel. I woke early, still simmering over the night before. 'I'll show him,' I thought to myself, as I scrawled a deliberately vague message dripping with melodrama and left it on the bedside table with. My. Phone. Sitting. Beside. It. The Drama! The Worry I would cause by leaving the flat – *gasp* – without my phone!

I marched down the four flights of stairs in triumph, and proceeded to wander around North London for a good two hours, topping up my feelings of self-righteousness by imagining what was going on two miles and four flights away:

- Tom moving through the stages of waking up (confusion),
- reading my note (irritation),
- calling my phone, only to hear it ringing inside the house (shock),
- then pacing our flat (four and a half paces across, so it would be quite quick pacing, but pacing nevertheless), finished by …
- blowing out from shame to worry to contrition to ABJECT DESPAIR.

After sitting on a bench in the churchyard for another hour, bum completely numb I finally headed home. I made sure to tiptoe up the stairs so I could hear his weeping over my sound of my footsteps. I opened the door slowly, eyes focusing down the hall …

… to see Tom still sound asleep, my note untouched and shuffling slightly in the breeze of his peaceful snoring.

Lesson #83: Don't play a hand you don't have.

What's next? Ah.

Lesson #84: Life is too short for bad lighting.

My mother taught me this early. The only time you should have the overhead lighting on in your home is if you're threading a needle, or suggesting people leave at the end of a party. Use lamps. Lots and lots of lamps. And don't trust a restaurant that lights your table like a gynaecologist's chair. They are serving you food, not peering into your nether regions. Smile, pay the bill, don't return.

Lesson #85: The onus of responsibility is on the communicator.

Emphasis mine. Heavy-handed, but necessary. Anyone who has worked for, or with, me has heard me say this too many times. It means *you* hold the responsibility of your burden, complaint, annoyance or grievance until you use your words to share it.

The other way we've discussed this rule in our house, is: 'use your words'. I have no time for passive aggression. Passive aggression is the chemical sweetener that poorly masks the taste of fury. Passive aggression is for people who hide behind curtains and etiquette. Passive aggression is for sad people too angry to use their words properly.

Lesson #86: You are better than passive aggression.

I suspect Virginia's mother-in-law was adept at 'using her words'. I never met Elizabeth (or Betty, as she was known), but I think I'd have liked her very much. Buzz explains what seems to be a typical interaction,

> *Early in our marriage [Betty] said to Virginia, 'You and Jim can come down to Laguna (they were retired at this stage) and bring*

the children. You will arrive at 11.00 am, we'll have lunch and you'll be gone by 3.00,' and Virginia said, 'Yes, Ma'am.'

What a wonderful invitation. I'd be there in a flash. And I'd be gone by 2.55 pm.

I certainly don't want anyone to think that I'm comparing Betty with a bull elephant – but if someone (or something) goes to the effort of providing clear instruction, it's polite to take notice. An experience of not leaving when prompted meant your grandmother and her parents nearly met a grisly end one afternoon in 1964. Buzz, Virginia and eleven-year-old Kate were touring around Amboseli National Park in Kenya, when they came across a huge elephant dozing in the midday sun. Grama starts off the story, that they all ended up sharing over the years:

It was while Buzz was driving … that he, Kate and I spotted the biggest bull elephant we'd ever seen. We edged the Volkswagen closer and closer across a dry lake bed to where he stood under a thorn tree. [We] then sat peering up at the six tons of scabby grey hide and brown streaked trunk. Buzz finished taking his elephant pictures and started the car, but when the [bull] heard the whine of the engine reversing, he suddenly came alive. With large ragged ears swung out and forward to focus on us, he pivoted on his massive hind legs and, with trunk outstretched and trumpeting, he charged! The only thing which saved us from his first lunge was Buzz shifting into forward gear thus changing direction as the elephant thundered past just behind us.

Or as my mother saw it:

Mum sits bolt upright and slaps the back of Dad's head [as he snapped photos], briskly as if she's testing a cantaloupe.

'Jim. JIM. I think that bull is getting ready to charge.'

Grama continues:

We set off cross country, the elephant right behind us. Kate and the lunch basket were thrown from one side of the back seat to the other. All Buzz could see in the rear view mirror was dust and tusks so he shouted, 'Is he still with us?'

Since I was trying to crawl under the seat I was in no position to investigate the situation and could only shriek, 'Yes, yes!'

When we were going almost thirty miles an hour the elephant finally dropped behind and it was then that Buzz decided to stop for one more picture. The elephant behaved beautifully, charged again, the central figure in a perfect action shot. I must admit I was not sharing Buzz's enthusiasm or, at this point, Kate's terror. I was just plain furious, yelling 'You bloody fool, get going!'

Mum again:

Now we are hurtling forward, bouncing like a toy. Nothing but red dust and tusks in the rear window. Then Mum does the most amazing thing. She swears at Dad, over and over and over again.

Buzz finishes the tale:

During this episode they were both lying on the floor calling me a bloody fool which I deserved. Anyway I have a marvellous photograph of this charging bull elephant.

Everybody who sees it asks, 'Oh, did you have a telephoto lens?'

I say, 'No, I didn't.'

Lesson #87: Always take the hint.

Other things you should keep in your car:

1. Dental floss.
2. A nail file.
3. Music. Singing loudly, singing passionately; singing the same lyrics over and over and over with no-one to tell you to turn it down or turn it off is one of life's purest pleasures.
4. Elephant repellant?

Lesson #88: Don't rely on others to help you leave.

Know how you'll leave and make sure you have the means to do so. This isn't just about getting out of bad parties before they get worse, this is about having an escape route from a toxic relationship or a poisonous job. I'm afraid, my darling, that this very often comes down to money. If you do not have enough, can I suggest applying for a credit card the very moment you have the means to, and then hiding it (literally) until – no, *unless* – you have no other way to get out. Your safety, physical and mental, is paramount. Everything else can be resolved. If you have to run and there's no-one else around remember that I'll be there, holding your hand.

There. That's that. Any more?

Lesson #89: If you don't ask, you won't know.

In 2018, you sat down and wrote a letter:

Dire Cwin,
Can I biy the princes
PS. Plis.

I will translate: 'Dear Queen, Can I Be The Princess? PS. Please.'

You waited patiently (and not so patiently) until one day, a heavy, creamy envelope arrived in our letterbox. A Lady, an actual lady-in-waiting, had replied to your letter! She told you that the Queen wished her to write to thank you for the colourful drawing and for your thoughtfulness.

I was charmed by the letter – hand-signed by Baroness Hussey, underneath the embossed logo, with the pleasingly formal prose.

You were confused and a little irritated that the Queen had neither made you a princess nor even acknowledged your request (which did confuse you). You decided to write again, but I'm not sure you did. Maybe it's best left alone, because if you haven't received a clear 'No', then maybe there is still the possibility of a 'Yes'?

Lesson #90: Sometimes, know when to stop asking.

Regardless of the outcome, my favourite part of this entire exchange is the 'PS. Please'.

Lesson #91: Manners are still important.

As I have said, you come from a long line of storytellers. And where you find a storyteller, you more than often find a reader. There's not much I can tell you about the glory and importance of reading that hasn't already been said, or that you don't already know. By the time you were eight your father and I had already had the distinct delight of watching you fall in love with reading. Gold medals may gather dust; certificates can fade on the wall. But the joy of seeing you head down in a book for the first time gave me the feeling that you'd summited a life pinnacle already.

You are a reader. What a superpower you have. Every book you have read will find a way to sit in your brain and rewire your neural pathways and pop out when you most need it.

When Jim was taking the long way to France across the United States, he wrote back to Kay:

> *... Going out to fight battles is what I've always dreamed of ever since I devoured [those adventure stories]... Even if I do fight greenish gas cylinders instead of glittering broadswords, the spirit is the same.*

Reading is the fuel to that imagination I told you about – the powerful tool that can help you through the very worst of things. Don't let anyone judge you on what books you read, and don't judge others for the same. Fiction, Politics, Raunchy rom-coms ... it doesn't matter. As long as people are absorbing the written word then you'll know they're a little bit more of 'your kind of person'.

> *Ella is learning to read,*
> *She hasn't developed much speed*
> *But give her the time,*
> *Be it fiction or rhyme,*
> *She will handle whatever they need.*
> *– K.G. and J.A. Quinby, 1984.*

Lesson #92: Never stop reading. Never stop writing.

Letter Thirteen

Discover the thrill of work

I resigned twice from my current job. The first time was even before I began working there, the second was the year I wrote these letters to you.

I had been diagnosed with cancer three days before starting a role at a Melbourne advertising agency in 2018. My new boss at the time didn't blink. 'Go do treatment, get better, and we'll be here waiting for you when you're ready.'

At the time I thought, 'This crazy Kiwi is never going to run a successful business if he keeps holding roles open for women dying of cancer.'

I was wrong on both counts.

Seven months later I put on a pair of heels for the first time since I'd been diagnosed and strode off to the pub to quit from that job I'd never started.

Both I and my Inner Monologue resigned: *I can't go back to ad-land! I'd had cancer!* Had? *I still probably have the damn thing! It's time to wrap myself in hemp clothing and meditate on a mountain for the rest of my life.*

The Kiwi Boss smiled, ordered a bottle of the Woodcutter's Shiraz and didn't take no for an answer.

Lesson #93: Hemp clothing and mountain-sitting can be boring, and don't tend to pay the bills.

And so I went to work. The agency sat within the shell of a nineteenth-century cable tram engineering shed. It had a red-brick facade from the 1890s, and a rooftop swimming pool from the 1980s. There, I found a team of clever and kind people who held me up and made me better while my body healed from treatment.

Rescinding that resignation was an excellent decision.

The second time I resigned from the same role was this year. I flew up from Victoria to New South Wales, masked and sanitised and thrilled at the banality of crossing the state line during a pandemic. We were in the middle of the exhausting throes of a global crisis and it was the first time I'd been allowed on a plane for over a year. It was Important. This time I was visiting another Boss: the Boss's Boss. Not a Kiwi this time, but also from another foreign country: Sydney.

There's a growing tendency in advertising agencies to do away with offices. Open plan is very chic. It's also impractical for private conversations like booking a leg wax, or resigning. When I walked through our head office and suggested to the Sydney boss that we'd 'need a room', I think he knew what was coming.

Both I and my Inner Monologue resigned: *'I can't stay in ad-land! I've signed a book contract! It's time to wrap myself in hemp clothing and use a typewriter for the rest of my life.'* He smiled and didn't take no for an answer. Which is how I'm writing this for you and still employed.

Lesson #94: When you do resign, do it face-to-face.

In advertising, they say, you're only one account-loss away from losing your job. To date, I've ended all my roles with resignations rather than redundancies. In this industry, this reflects very little on me and a lot on luck. It also means that after delivering four 'Dear John' letters over fifteen years, I have two rules for resignation. The first is above, the second, below:

Lesson #95: The best time to leave a job is when you feel you're not quite ready.

Work – in advertising at least – can be thrilling. Like a great love affair it makes you glow, while also casting its light on everything else around you. When work is good, everything is good. Also like an affair, when it's bad – it's very, very horrid. I have had great jobs, I have had terrible ones. The difference? Mostly me.

I started my earning life with jobs in Melbourne as soon as I was allowed. A teenager moving through restaurants, department stores, nannying jobs and call centres. We've already discussed how some of these went a good way to teaching me about the jerks of the world. Yet they were still middle-class jobs of privilege. Which is how I thought my Grama started out her working life as well. Until I came to the part about the jar of cold cream in a sock:

> *Every year from the age of fourteen I worked in a variety of summer jobs. At first they consisted of garden maintenance for people on vacation. I'd ride my bike over to the job of the day where I'd weed and water for fifteen cents an hour. The pay was marginally better for later summer jobs I held, such as nurse's aide in the Stanford Hospital, mail girl for a San Francisco insurance company and matron at Santa Clara County Juvenile Detention Home in San Jose. The position had previously been held by a friend but she had been injured on duty and no longer wanted the job.*

'Injured' doesn't really cover it:

One of the girls being detained in Juvenile Hall had sat on top of an open door, waiting for the matron to pass through. When she did she was hit by a cold cream jar in a sock.

After leaving school, Virginia went from her student role as Matron to a full-time one as Deputy Juvenile Probation Officer. The job was tough; she was twenty-three and grappling with foster families, adoptions and abuse. Buzz said of his new wife's posting:

It wasn't a nice job – she was handling kids with cigarette burns on their backs, placing them in foster homes. Also handling teenagers and she was only twenty-three herself. They were a hard bunch some of those teenagers – she used to take them down to the correctional center in Los Angeles in the county car and by the time she [returned] they were already back in San Jose.

None of my early jobs included cigarette burns or besocked jars of moisturiser. But assault doesn't need to be involved for it to be a difficult first job. Nevertheless, if it's okay with you, I'd prefer if your jobs actively avoid any violence.

The jobs I've had taught me things. They taught me how not to be a jerk, as you know. They also taught me how to carve friendships out in the most difficult of circumstances. They taught me how to experience self-worth in a way a romance couldn't (and most certainly shouldn't). They taught me to see taxes as inevitable. Well, almost inevitable.

Before beginning her career in advertising, Mum was at art school and needed to pay rent. She and her mate ran the flower cart on Dandenong Road. It was 1976:

We set up the cart by 6.30, and De Groot delivers the flowers by 7.00. The disco-tragics are pulling up in taxis, even before the bunches are out in buckets.

[By the end of the day] we never have any flowers left, though I often think it would be nice to take some home.

I count the cash while Judy goes to the car. She hitches the cart up, we get in and stuff the wads of notes into our tiny jeans. We unzip them first, and lie back to pull the zips up again.

When that's sorted we go to the pub. We pay no tax and never bother applying for a hawker's licence. Hell, we don't even buy our own drinks. We buy our own houses instead.

As soon as I graduated from university I started working full time, and Mum charged me board. It was considerably less than I would have been paying if I'd moved out of home, but it still made a statement from her and an impression on me. Later, as London plans gathered steam, I requested that I continue to pay her the money but she divert it into my 'London' savings account for six months. She agreed, and privilege continued to follow me.

Lesson #96: Acknowledge your privilege.

My first job in London was via a temp agency called Office Angels. The logo was pink and had a halo. They fed us free takeaway lunches on Fridays.

They placed me in my first role on reception at a quantity surveyors on Holyrood Street, tucked down a laneway that felt very Jack the Ripper-y, even in the stinking summer months I worked there. That heatwave I'd arrived in was simmering on. Thirty degrees in London is not like thirty degrees in Melbourne. Its grip is tighter, slimier, sweatier and smellier. It's the heat of an old city that's never touched the ocean, and hasn't yet managed to befriend air-conditioning. The office was so hot that I'd stand in the loos running cold water over my upturned wrists. They must have thought I had a stomach complaint.

On my first day I sat at the desk, the only woman in the twelve-person office. The phone rang.

'Canah speyt ta-ian i'accounts, it's 'ob.'

Shit.

'Er, yes – um, sorry. Can you please repeat that?'

'Its 'obmorty – ah need Ian.'

Ian. Ian Ian.

'Putting you through!' My armpits started to prickle with anxiety.

When I was told at the end of that first morning that I needed to actually pass the caller's details on when I was connecting the call, the anxiety prickle spread up into my chest as a stress rash.

I had no idea what any of these people were saying.

'Helloa theear – it's Michael fra Yorkshabank, can ah call ta Nigel.'

Shit. Shit.

'Putting you through!' Cheerfully, madly punching buttons. 'Erm, Nigel? It's … (swallows) Michael-fra-York-sha-bank?' It didn't sound right with my upward-Aussie inflection. I held my breath, waiting for Nigel to ask me what the hell I was saying.

'Thank you Ella, put him through.'

*

As Jim moved through Europe, he could observe a wider range of accents than he had in his home country.

> *We learned, in that business, to distinguish the types of speech of the different nationalities, at a distance, even when the individual words could not be distinguished. When Germans talk, it's [a guttural sound]. When Frenchmen talk, it [is a] fluttering sound, higher-pitched. And when Americans talk, they grumble for awhile and then swear.*

Moving to another country that speaks your language is diving into a pool, only to find it's a river. Already speaking the language tricks you into thinking everything else is the same as it is at home. You are lulled into a sense of safety because you can understand the tannoy on the airport shuttle, and can read the signs on the Underground.

Both Virginia and Buzz had their own challenges during that first overseas posting in Melbourne. You'll recall that they had arrived from sunny California to a grey, conservative city sitting at least two decades behind the country they had left. And no-one it seemed, spoke American:

> *Jim was fast learning the ropes at the office. It wasn't easy. When the phone on his desk rang for the first time he couldn't understand the garbled speech on the other end. He exchanged the 'faulty instrument' for a new one but it, too, was unintelligible. Not the telephone but Jim's ear was the problem and he gradually grew to understand the accent coming over the line.*

Virginia's own experience wasn't much easier, but she didn't have a telephone to blame her ear on:

> *'Toolenhaypnymisermum?' answered one pleasant woman when I asked the price of an item. Baffled by her accent I had to ask her again and after the third time I understood, paid her two shillings and eleven pence halfpenny and told her I didn't miss my mother very much.*

Lesson #97: It's not quite so much what you say, but what you hear.

For all of the time I worked in Holyrood Street, I phonetically repeated every call I received, never knowing who I was talking to, or what about. But I didn't get fired. Instead, they paid me –

real British pounds! With my first payslip I went back to the list I had written in that homesick cafe. After my bills, I bought a can of hairspray, a magazine and flowers for the Top Floor Flat.

After the second payslip, I bought a pair of kitten heels that I'd been coveting from a candy-striped shop in Covent Garden. I only ever wore them inside and *never* on the cobblestones, so they lasted and lasted. I still own those shoes with their buttersoft leather.

I'm telling you these things not because buying shit is important, but being able to buy the shit you want, with your own money, is really important. Your great-great-grandmother discovered this when she went to Washington to assist the war effort:

> *On the 21st of August 1918 [my friend Alice and I] set out for the nation's capital with great enthusiasm and a zest for adventure. The city in wartime was a fascinating place and my salary of $1000.00 a year seemed quite adequate. Housing was difficult but after a short stay at Ingleside Terrace, where we barricaded the bedroom door against possible intruders, we found a good room with a family in Georgetown. It was an exciting winter. By economizing on the essentials we had money enough for theater tickets, sight-seeing and trips to New York.*

Lesson #98: Earn your independence.

When the Office Angels placed me elsewhere, the men at the Quantity Surveyors took me for lunch at a pub with peanut shells on the floor and said thank you.

At least, I think that's what they said.

*

I did not like temping. It gave me all the worst bits about an office job (the fluoro lighting, the awkward kitchenette-chat, the emails about toilet habits) without any of the good bits (paid annual leave, the intimacy of spending hard times with clever people, the emails about toilet habits).

After the quantity surveyors' office I moved to the 'General Social Care Council', a now-defunct government agency with a multimillion pound view of the Thames. It was a job that paid well and ended at 4.55 pm every day, when the entire floor of workers simultaneously stood up and began putting on their coats – like choreographed meerkats. On my first day of this performance I was still gawping at my desk when the last employee exited into the lift and left me alone, solo in a floor of blinking PC monitors. It was a seamless departure of puffer jackets and rucksacks. When I asked after this mass migration the next morning, it was explained to me that everyone ensured they left their desks at 4.55 pm so they'd be out on the street at their contractually agreed time of 5 pm.

I resolved never to work in a job where the clock dictated my commitment. Which is lucky, because that was the same year I pulled my first all-nighter in a job.

I temped in London for six months while I tried to find my 'proper' job. Old notebooks show names of friends of friends and receptionist email addresses and A–Z Map references of agencies down side streets and atop shiny glass buildings. A word-map of trying, trying, trying. Nowadays they call it 'hustle', but back then I just ... persisted. Sitting in various receptions across Soho and East London, cold-eyed assistants and enormous floral arrangements (lilies, always lilies). Linking one conversation to the next, waiting and hoping for a home.

I found one, in a 'little' agency that by my Melbourne standards seemed enormous. In an odd way, it ended up curing my first prick of homesickness, because no-one knew anything about Australia, and no-one knew anything about me.

It was wonderful. The office was in an old toffee factory in the backstreets near Euston Station. A tiny caff on the nearby Georgian terrace was called 'Wot the Dickens' and sold mayonnaise, tuna and sweetcorn sandwiches. I was almost faint with delight at the Britishness of it all. There was a dance academy next door, so our office windows often looked onto collections of dancers stretching themselves and their various limbs on balconies and terraces and lampposts. The vast basement delivered hot staff lunches every day, served up by Rosie, a much-loved cook who was the first person I heard say the word 'motherfucker' in the workplace.

Everything about the agency was foreign and every minute of that initial year working was filled with the electric fizz of firsts. My first proper advertising agency. My first group of London-made and London-built friends. My first expenses claim. My first snowfall, spied through those rippled Georgian glass windows, onto the cobbled street. My first all-nighter on a pitch, sleeping on a sofa in the attic offices and brushing my teeth as the cleaners arrived. My first understanding that work can be home when your home is very far away. My first time flirting with one person while living with another.

That job was the beginning of my entire life.

Lesson #99: Your first proper job will always be your best.

After three years, I left the toffee factory. I left because I was getting, as I explained at the time, 'fat and happy'. Which I think is a mid-twenties way of saying, 'I don't think I can write the same email over and over for another three years.' Or, alternatively, 'I'd like more money and shinier offices and bigger boardrooms.' What I didn't realise is the latter had no bearing on the former.

It was my first big lesson in being careful what you wish for. I moved to another London ad agency and another factory. It felt right that I was leaving the comfort of the old toffee factory for the disquiet of the old cigarette factory guarded by those enormous black cats. It was an office of hundreds of people, and every day there was a different pair of feet weeping in a toilet stall.

Lesson #100: The more 'successful' the company, the more likely you'll hear weeping in the loos.

There was a team-bonding exercise at that black cat agency. We had to get together and make an enormous, oversized version of food: 'Pimp My Snack'-style. Our group was allocated 'sushi'. I have no memory of the sushi itself, but the presentation afterward involved us setting up a laptop to play the making-of film to the entire department. As is always the case, the tech failed. The half-dozen or so of our group sat stiff in our seats while the most junior member of Team Sushi tried in vain to fix the issue up on the stage. None of us got up to help. I remember how hot with referred embarrassment my face was, how much I didn't want to go up there with the flame-red blush to help repair it, and how I blushed even harder when the department lead later called the group out on it.

'You left her to sort it all on her own. You stood by and watched.'

She was right. It was a shitty thing to do and it was my own immaturity that allowed me to do it. It was a lesson learned that day. A lesson to fix your own tech, collect your own dry cleaning, and never – ever – leave a member of the team out there on their own.

Lesson #101: One in, all in.

As an officer, Jim had the most extreme of team-bonding exercises. In, you know, a world war:

> *I dug my own foxhole, by the way, basically because I wanted it dug right. I wanted it the right size for me. I carried my own shovel; I dug my own foxhole … because I couldn't fix the responsibility of digging mine on one man; that wouldn't be fair. Besides, if an officer does his own work, he's more popular with the men, and he isn't as likely to get shot in the back.*

Lesson #102: Carry your own shovel, and dig your own foxhole.

I found another work-home back in Melbourne, not in a disused factory this time, but a disused department store. Beginning in 2007, I was there for almost a decade. Late in my tenure – years after Georges' department store had closed – we'd still have confused old ladies emerging from the elevator into reception, asking where the haberdashery department was.

Elevators still ran between floors, where original department listings remained on the lifts' walls. Although in our residency we used them as recording booths for rough voiceovers. The creative teams would throw a few cushions on the floor of the lift. With the doors closed, the acoustics were perfect.

It was a marvellous building, filled with people humming at the thrill of doing some of the best work of their career so far. The creative output was epic and the parties were legendary. Or was it the other way around? Either way, Friday night drinks in the office bar often turned into parties better than any I'd ever thrown (or, let's be honest, attended).

At the end of another week of making ads, we all tried, merrily, to kill ourselves. A dumbwaiter ran between the old staff canteen kitchen and the Georges' 'executive boardroom' on the floor below. Some of the smaller members of staff rode the dumbwaiter up and down while we raced them via the wide stone internal staircase.

Victorian windows high above Collins Street were jacked open and we all hung too-far out of them, waving cigarettes and drinks at the crowds exiting the Regent and Atheneum theatres, floors below. Health, safety, what's that? We were young, dumb and full of advertising.

*

My grandfather actually worked in an elevator once – a step up from a dumbwaiter, but still, an elevator:

> *Buzz's [New York] office, he told me, was a disused elevator. It had no window and when the door closed it did so with the ominous *whush* of an airlock. He never invited me to visit that office. He wasn't proud of this stage of his career. He wasn't happy.*

Buzz wasn't happy. This isn't abnormal. There are times when a job is shit. I've had terrible bosses, lazy colleagues and nasty clients. I've been in over my head and way out of my depth and drowning between the two. Sometimes, something doesn't click. The job may be too hard, too easy, or just too far away. The trick is not to avoid these jobs, because it's very hard to establish what's wrong until you're in the thick of it. The trick is to identify what's wrong once you're in the middle of the wrong.

Some people felt about the cigarette factory the way I felt about the toffee factory or the department store. And vice versa. Often, it's not the workplace that's wrong, it's who you are at the time you work there. In my time at the toffee factory I was falling in love, both with advertising and with a man. Behind those black cats, I was homesick, hungry and tired. In my time in the department store, I was growing a career and a friendship group and a marriage.

Lesson #103: If you can't change you, and you can't change them, change jobs.

The one thing I want to tell you more than anything is – find a job that makes you better. Don't be better than the job, it's the quickest way to breed resentment and dull your own blade. Find a job that excites you, scares you, lifts you up, educates you and makes you laugh. Find a job where the people you do the work with are as good as (or better than) the work itself. I think you and I both know what I'm saying here, my girl …

Lesson #104: Your job is what you make it.

Go get 'em.

Letter Fourteen

Smells

Back to dying. If our taste goes first, I believe the next sense to disappear is smell. Which is good, because hospitals – where most of us will die – tend to smell of antiseptic and fear. But it's also sad because, between Virginia and Kate and me, scent takes up a disproportionate amount of the detail we love and remember.

Here's Grama, at the beginning of 1960 and the beginning of her first travels through Asia:

> *The impact of Singapore was so sharp I could taste the smells. Laundry hung from poles over narrow lanes, monkeys squabbled for our bananas in the Botanic Gardens, snake charmers and pedicabs waited outside our hotel.*

And then my mum, eleven years old in 1964 and spending her Saturday at a Kenyan riding school:

> *Horse poo, hay and red clay dust. I love this smell.*

Putting laundry and red clay dust aside, if we're talking about smells, we could start with flowers. In this family, they come tumbling and falling and straining up through dirt. But that's too obvious. Every family has flowers.

Let's begin with artichokes; the urea-green smell of boiled artichokes. That's better. That will be one of our base notes. We're making a scent, did I say? And from the little I know, some of the most famous scents contain indelicate sources: deer musk, whale poo, even human sweat. But don't worry, our scent will be absolutely delightful and it may even come in a special glass bottle with a heavy stopper that goes 'clunk' when it is replaced.

If we were to mix a family scent, it would most certainly have notes of artichoke. I smelt it first as a child, during quiet weekend afternoons at home. Mum cooked them on the stove long enough for the glass of the back room windows to fog up. Or maybe that was the tumble dryer going? The tumble dryer didn't smell of artichoke, though. Sunday was laundry and artichoke day. We'd eat the latter after the chores were complete, sharp leaves flipped over and dragged along bottom teeth. Dipped into American mayonnaise, which back then could only be procured by driving out to the USA Food Store, a beacon to homesick Yanks, sitting incongruously between business parks and industrial estates. It was far enough out of Melbourne that anything purchased beneath the red, white and blue flag had to be rationed. Artichoke day was a special day.

Winter weekends often fog up our own windows as well, in this house that we live in now, and that you moved into when you were just over one year old. I often sag into our couch on a Sunday night, body tired from the hours of administration it takes to weekend in a middle-class Melbourne family. It's then that I think of my mother. The two days that Tom and I share is forty-eight hours of lists. Garden, laundry, bills, family, repairs, friends, animals, more laundry. Mum had to work through it all alone. I wasn't aware of her solo-ness when I was that young, but in hindsight (always in hindsight) I consider her and her isolation as she moved through the loads of clothes, the bills paid by chequebook at the kitchen table, the mowing of the lawn, the sewing of name tags on school uniforms, the packed lunches in brown paper bags. It creates a feeling that my grandmother inadvertently put into words for me:

> *Only as an adult did I realise that those years were not without worries …*

Every Sunday Mum visits Grama in her nearby Point Lonsdale nursing home. Before leaving, Mum boils up artichokes and takes them in a Tupperware container along with other Rich Gifts (a *Time* magazine, a block of Old Gold Rum n Raisin chocolate, a takeaway coffee). Together they sit in Grama's bedroom – that last bedroom: a single bed, a little further from the sea. There is no shingled roof or frosted lampshade, but it's cosy and has that hand-sewn quilt on the bed. It is, as Grama would say, a 'solitary and untroubled existence':

> *What a solitary and untroubled existence I led during my preschool years. Hours spent playing with Teddy and my doll Nana on the kitchen floor while Mother ironed and the boiling artichokes added their fragrance to the aroma of freshly pressed pillowcases. Only as an adult did I realise that those years were not without worries for my parents.*

Grama was born in 1927. As her father said, 'coming along at the same time as the Depression did'. It wasn't until I discovered the above passage that I realised she has been eating artichokes all her life.

Artichokes smell of wee, and seaweed smells of the sea. But overripe sea. Sea that doesn't belong on land.

The smell of seaweed saved the life of Buzz, once. As an officer in the US Navy, he on was shore leave in Qingdao (then called Tsingtao), China, in 1944, and had ventured to the local Marine

Officer's Club by the beach. Buzz had a little .32 calibre pistol that his then-fiancée's father had given him before he deployed. He holstered it and went for drinks. When Buzz emerged from the club, the rest of his officer group hailed pedicabs and left ahead of him. So he jumped into the one remaining rickshaw, which started off suspiciously slowly. Buzz and his driver quickly dropped behind. He started to yell, but the rickshaw driver pretended not to hear him. Buzz said,

> *I could tell we were getting further and further away from the water because I couldn't smell the seaweed any longer.*
>
> *It was darker than hell and all of a sudden we went into this courtyard. [The driver] flicked the rickshaw over, I did a roll and came up with the gun out. I could just see these characters standing there with some knives. They were going to rob or kill me. [Then], they saw the gun and they left. So, there I was … back walking towards where I thought the beach was.*

Artichokes smell of wee and seaweed smells of the sea, and I'm glad for Buzz's fiancée, Audrey. He didn't marry her, but he did manage to frighten off a bunch of knife-wielding characters in a Chinese port thanks to her, her father and that little pistol.

Lesson #105: Keep your nostrils open, as well as your eyes.

Shall we talk about flowers now? We can't avoid them for much longer. They're everywhere in our family tapestry. We love a good petal-wafted smell, we do. Grama's parents were avid gardeners, and her childhood garden was lush and overgrown:

> *The impressive orchard contained not only the plum tree which was to hold my treehouse, but cherry, apricot, peach, almond, pear, fig, nectarine and apple trees. Mother was soon kept busy canning the fruit in Mason jars. Lilac and heliotrope, roses and*

nicotiana were planted outside bedroom windows to scent our dreams. And mock orange, a flower which brings an aching, nameless yearning when I smell it now. Beyond the syringa in the back yard was a row of Copper Queens, single roses which glowed red-orange.

I had to Google most of those flowers, to my great shame. My floral knowledge is a little more basic: gardenia, daphne, nasturtiums and frangipani. I do recognise one thing with deep familiarity though: that aching, nameless yearning.

There is a large daphne bush planted at the front step of number 38 and its budded tips pump out scent midwinter. There was daphne at Jim and Kay's house, too, and maybe that's why Mum planted her own bush at her own threshold. I still bend down and inhale every time I walk past during a blooming month. This is normally July, when the Melbourne winter is feeling like it's settled in our bones and will never leave. That daphne burst is an early flag that spring is coming and soon the moss and leaf litter will give way to wattle pollen, and not long afterwards – temperamental gardenia.

Your Gaga has been wearing a gardenia scent for much of my life. I already know the smell of it will make me sob once she's gone.

Lesson #106: Wear a scent, and make it your own.

The most common reason for me to go back to number 38 nowadays is to collect you. Mum picks you up from school twice a week, but when you were younger she had you for two full days. It is a primal feeling to receive your child at the end of a day and smell your own mother on her skin. A primal feeling and a particular privilege.

When you were born, your breath smelt of caramel. We'll add that. As well as throwing in the daphne and the gardenia. All of those will go into the pot. Stir, stir, stir. It'll be too sweet soon – we need some spice. Nasturtium petals taste of pepper and smell similarly, as Grama would've found when she was young and vacationing with her family in a borrowed beach house:

> *This white stucco English style cottage stood on the cliff-top facing Carmel Bay. Monterey cypresses crowded in round the house, adding their scent to that of seaweed and salt. The house would smell damp and musty after being closed for long periods and I'd be sent out to pick the fragrant nasturtiums that tumbled down the cliff face. Bowls of their orange and yellow flowers and windows open to the stiff breeze soon aired the rooms.*

Nasturtiums also tumbled around the back garden of Shenzi. That's where Grama taught me to pinch the ends off the funnel-shaped spur beneath the orange and yellow petals and sip the sweet nectar. I always felt a little naughty, as if I were stealing from the fairies' larder. I taught you to do the same with the nasturtiums in our garden – with the added step in the ritual of peering into the spur to ensure there are no hidden ants. You are still very strict about this. I guess this is after an occasion of drinking more ant than nectar.

Gardenia is Mum, daphne is Home, nasturtiums are Grama and frangipani is Joy. Creamy petals that narrow into a yellow blush, frangipanis smell of tropical nights on our tiny Fijian island where we are always happy. They were less exotic to Mum, who clambered over them in the mid-1960s when she, Grama, Buzz and the rest of their family lived in Accra, Ghana:

> *Behind the bougainvillea hedge glowed a bed of gerberas, so common in Africa that their jewel colours went unnoticed. The front circular drive was edged with low hedges and curved past frangipani trees so large the children could climb them.*

Flowers! We've enough. What else? Something stronger, darker – how about smoke? We know that Kay wore Bourjois' 'Evening in Paris' and that Jim smelt of tobacco and ivory soap. We know this because Kate smelt that on her Grampa when dancing in their living room, and I smelt Big Grampa's pipe when I visited at age thirteen. He had been gone some years by then, but it still smelt warm and rough and wise.

On a similar vein (or as perfumers call it, 'the base notes'), let's add the yeast of Victoria Bitter and the nuttiness of salted peanuts. This is the smell of my father after a day at work. It's comforting and warm and very far away, like most childhood memories.

And there is also the scent of a 1980s ad agency on the weekend. I would trail into the office after Dad while he collected or completed something. As he was busy I would potter around the floor, dim in the after-hours, the fluorescent lights switched off, the air-conditioning units still. An advertising agency before desktop computers existed smelt of spray-mount glue, Pantone ink, cigarettes from the studio's overflowing ashtrays and the *sillage* of 'Pino Silvestre' aftershave. Let's take a drop of the ink and leave the rest be.

Lesson #107: If you can smell your scent five minutes after application, you're wearing too much.

We have flowers and perfume and ink, but should we add the smallest chemical drop of gas? It is pungent, but to Kay represented a magical window into a new world of possibility. She writes of these childhood days in the very early years of the twentieth century:

> *The orange ranch which my father bought in Santa Ana was also a good place for a child and I remember with pleasure the house built by my parents ... In the front ... was a large screened-in porch and it was here that I saw my first home movies projected by a machine which a client had given my father.*

It had an acetylene lamp which made a rasping noise and had a most unpleasant smell. There were two reels of film, one of girls diving off a diving board and one of men cutting trees in a forest. It was all such a novelty that we ran the pictures over and over again.

What about something green? Woody and warm? With a family who have spent almost three generations with thousands of miles separating loved ones, we are good at using scent as a missive across the oceans. When Buzz and Virginia were bringing children up far away from their grandparents, Jim and Kay would send Christmas gifts from California to wherever they were stationed: Australia, Africa, New Zealand – home always made its way. Often, Virginia tells us, there would be a 'spray of California redwood laid across the gift-wrapped parcels inside to give us a whiff of home'.

Christmas is where so many smells make their homes in recollection. I remember Mum, in the years thick with single-motherdom, creating a Christmas-scented memory as only an advertising creative with three decades of experience under her belt can do. We would have a plastic Christmas tree, as it was easier for her to put up and take down on her own. The smell was missing, though.

So one Christmas, she approached our local greengrocer (in the days when Bridport Street still held shops for shopping, rather than for browsing). Mum asked the fruiterer if he had any Christmas tree offcuts.

'Of course!' In my memory he had a broad face and fingers that pinched my cheeks. I called him Mister Poggi.

Mum marched home with boughs of sap-tacky Monterey pine in her arms, and dropped them, hidden, behind the couch in the front room. All Christmas long people exclaimed as they entered the house, 'Oh Kate, your tree smells divine!' When we told them it was plastic they never believed us.

Lesson #108: Scent is more powerful than sight.

We need something to finish off our scent. I could choose so many, so many smells that hit me in the limbic system and take me back in time with brutal efficiency:

The insipid toilet freshener in a job that was relentlessly grinding me down, unpicking years of self-worth and experience.

The stringency of alcohol wipes from the IVF days, when I stuck myself with more needles than a pin cushion.

The hollow chemical smell of my portable chemo balloon, hung around my neck like a poisonous albatross that also happened to be killing my cancer.

No, let's leave those off the table.

A final scent will be added. Wet wood.

Bear with me – it's distinct and subtle but I've experienced it twice in two different parts of the world. When we were staying in that palatial Puglian *masseria* and that dusky-voiced chef ushered us out to the deck for dinner, the smell of the timber we walked over was so powerfully evocative that I felt dizzy with space and time travel. It was exactly that of the hot decking out the back of Shenzi, around Buzz's home-installed above-ground swimming pool. The timber dark with water, wet down by the hose and splintering our bums as we slid into the water. Point Lonsdale to Italy. Eight years old to twenty-four. By that maths, the next time I'm due to walk over sun-drenched wet wood is this coming year, my fortieth. When I find it I'll drop it into the pot. Stir, stir, stir.

Let's call the scent 'Recollection'. Or 'Nostalgia'.

Or simply: 'Everything'.

Letter Fifteen

Bleeding

Life with a uterus is a life of bleeding. It is the uncertain beginning of bleeding, it is pretending we are not bleeding, it is the hushed cessation of bleeding.

And it is the expectation that throughout we bleed, and smile. And smile, and bleed.

This is a letter about my bits, and the role my bits have played in my life. Which, I get isn't what you may want from your mother today. Yet there will come a time when you *are* interested. When you *do* want to know. And that is what this letter is for.

When you're being pursued by a pissed-off mountain lion, you don't stop to worry about the blisters you might get running away. This is how it felt when I was told my cancer treatment would cause early menopause. I was sitting in my radiotherapist's office having the Talk. The one in which they impress upon you how serious your cancer is, and how important your treatment is, and how there may be side-effects to that treatment.

We didn't discuss the specifics in that appointment. Instead, we talked about the likelihood that I might die if I didn't start treatment urgently. I was okay with this approach. I wasn't thinking of the side-effects either. I was thinking of you, five years old, playground-bruised knees and a missing tooth, and how I would wrestle one hundred raging mountain lions if it meant I would be alive on the other side.

I was also pleased to be having this conversation with this particular specialist, because he had used the word 'vulva' and 'cervix' while maintaining eye contact. Which seems expected for a doctor, but, unfortunately, is not.

Not long before that, your father and I were auditioning my treatment team. It was like *Australian Idol*, but with more brochures and whispering. Earlier that week we had met a prospective radiotherapist in a glossy office. I stuck my hand out, ready to shake. He reciprocated, but held only the tips of my fingers. Some might say gently, but I was in a prickly mood (I'd just been diagnosed with cancer after all). I felt he was treating me like a fragile girl-doll with girl-cancers in my girl-body. It wasn't a great beginning.

When we asked pointed questions, the specialist said my radiation treatment would feel like 'a bad sunburn' and my pain 'might get a little challenging'. His manner creased my brow. It also set my advertising-attuned bullshit-meter dinging.

The doctor waved towards my PET scan on his computer screen, the multiple malignancies glowing white like a spider's egg sacs. A scan that among other organs showed my ovaries, uterus and cervix. When he did so, he referred to them as, 'Your … *ahem* … lady parts.'

Oh dear. Tom could barely usher me out of the room before I started sputtering and gesticulating.

The next day we were with another specialist in another cancer department in another hospital. This is the one who made eye contact with me. He also used the correct terminology for my organs, which is a plus for a medical professional.

We asked the same questions, but he used different language. He told us the treatment and its side-effects would be 'brutal', and that hospitalisation for pain management would be 'vital'.

'By the time I finish with you, you'll wish you'd never met me.' Which is right, but wrong too – because he helped save my life.

Lesson #109: Trust your gut.

Two years after that treatment finished I received the call from my GP confirming I was 'in menopause'. Which sounds like a terrible place to be, at any time of day.

My daughter, I'm not proud to admit how winded I felt on hearing this news. Because enough time had passed since those mountain lion days. Those just-diagnosed days when the hollow fear of mortality allowed me to mean it when I said, 'I don't care what happens, just let me survive.'

'What happens' was more tangible by the time I got that phone call. And menopause sounded disappointing and dusty. Maybe it's my vanity, but the very word felt like someone had scrubbed out big chunks of my person. I felt less female, less powerful, less attractive, less strong. I just felt *less*.

Virginia was thirty-four when she had a hysterectomy in the 1960s.

That she's even committed this to paper is something, whereas I've struggled to do the same:

> *Problems followed [my youngest's] birth. After eight weeks my postnatal bleeding hadn't stopped and I thought a hysterectomy would be a good idea. [My doctor] didn't entirely agree. He felt surgery would be unnecessarily drastic and that it was too soon after my baby's birth. I begged.*
>
> *Finally he said, 'You're a very persuasive woman. Alright, I'll perform the surgery.'*
>
> *My neighbour, who had had the same operation a year before, was just the friend I needed at that time and could answer all the silly questions I couldn't ask [the doctor]. She even drove me to the Bowen Street Hospital the day before surgery.*

There's a lot here, not least Grama's use of the term 'silly questions'. In this context, Dr Lady Parts makes more sense. He was not a bad doctor, he was just an old one. His language was better suited to another time. Maybe, to Grama's time.

Regardless, I can't think of any scenario in this day in which a postnatal woman would convince a doctor to perform a hysterectomy. But clearly it wasn't too strange if Virginia's neighbour had had the same operation. Grama doesn't go into the detail of how she felt afterwards, besides her 'tender incision', but there is a description of the challenging time during her recovery when Christmas was rolling on – seemingly – without her.

> *I was released from the hospital a few days before Christmas, weak and shaky. Back at [home] I crawled into bed, gazed up at the looming black wardrobe and felt it was going to be an awful Christmas. Nothing would be done correctly, in our traditional way. We were so lucky to have Alice [a housekeeper] but the stuffing she was planning for the turkey didn't sound like my stuffing. I felt dispossessed. The rest of the family was happy and busy with their own preparations. Even Jim didn't seem to understand how left out I felt.*

Darling, am I being too much of a university student in first year Feminist Studies to correlate Virginia's feeling of being dispossessed of her Christmas to Virginia feeling dispossessed of something else?

> *[Alice] cooked a perfect Christmas dinner and her son joined us for a happy, happy day. In the afternoon Jim helped me into the car and we drove across the street for drinks with the neighbours. Only a fifteen-minute stay but it gave me the feeling I wasn't an isolated invalid. Jim did understand.*

Menopause feels like another badge I should proudly pin to my twenty-first century Equality Uniform. I am proud to call myself a feminist. But menopause? Menopause isn't something discussed at the dinner table. Not even ours. I may be a woman who Instagrammed her bum cancer, but in the early days I could barely say the 'M' word aloud to your father without flinching. Because even in this time of growing enlightenment, I thought menopause needed to be suffered through.

Going through early menopause at thirty-six meant, much like the inducement of labour, I never knew what it felt like to naturally move into the next stage of my reproductive life. It hit me hard. I experienced 'hot flushes' and 'night sweats' like they should be named: 'scalding hives' and 'insomniac drenchings'. My belly became rotund in a way even pregnancy hadn't reshaped. My skin, my hair, my mind: everything changed. Yet even then I – the person who seeks medical reassurance like others pop out for a coffee – dragged my feet to see the specialist.

Because I chalked the misery of every symptom up to vanity and flippancy. Instead of seeing a doctor, I asked myself questions.

'How could night sweats be life-threatening?'

'Why am I so pathetically obsessed with my newly round stomach?'

'Why is "gunt" such an angry, ugly word?'

My period was something I got young: in 1992, at eleven years old. Which meant for twenty-five years I bled, cramped and clotted my way through a week in every month. I don't miss my period. It was tedious, inconvenient, and – when we were trying to get pregnant – a monthly blot of failure on white toilet paper. Despite all this, having stashes of tampons in office drawers and moaning about monthly cravings anchored me in a demographic I felt comfortable in.

I left that demographic and all it contained behind with thirty sessions of pelvic radiation. My little shrivelled ovaries: I picture them like sad raisins.

It's acceptable to moan about periods because they're something that almost half of us have for over half of our lives. A little flag of fertility that even if we don't choose to wave, we *might*. Then why couldn't I moan about menopause? Why so quiet?

Back in the antique years of the 1990s, Menstruation and Menopause were taught as the two bookmarks of 'womanhood'. But in the time that has passed between my first period and your first school anatomy lesson, the world has opened up. Just a little, like a flower with an angle more light and a drop more water – something is growing. A quiet blossoming of awareness, support and understanding about gender, sexuality and identity, and how the physical self connects to all of this.

You as a nine-year-old seem to have a more profound understanding of these things than I did ten years ago. Which is wonderful. This is what improvement is all about. If my daughter – you – can understand that identity is not tied to physicality, then why can't I? Why did the medical declaration of my menopause feel like such an attack on my womanhood? Why, my girl, was I so quiet?

Lesson #110: Menopause is a feminist issue.

I think it's because to acknowledge menopause is to also acknowledge what it takes away. For some women, it asserts the absence of qualities we are meant to have, but mustn't admit directly to coveting: youth, elasticity, composure, sexuality, tranquillity. To feel the loss of any of these is to reveal you enjoyed them in the first place. Which – in my experience – is the very opposite of how a serene woman must act. She 'must' inhabit youth and verve, but incidentally, rather than in an ardent way.

This woman must wear the jewels of femininity across her hands, wrists and ears – but never be seen to admire them, to never be observed watching them dance and twinkle in the sun.

Lesson #111: *Wear your jewels and be proud of them.*

This is a letter about blood and it is also a letter about the burden your sex and your gender may place upon you. It's about some of the burdens the women who walked before you carried. Mostly, it's about the micro-burdens we have all sustained, without knowing it.

The journey of a woman who is paid to work begins with a 'Before' and ends with an 'After'. *Before* I had a child. *After* I had a child. Before I had a child I worked as long as I wanted without any consequence. After I had a child, I watched single parents in my office and wondered how they managed to survive. How did any of us survive? American journalist and podcaster Amy Westervelt succinctly wrapped up all our 'After' feelings when she said, 'We expect women to work like they don't have children, and raise children as if they don't work.'

Kate, my own single mother, survived as long and as hard as she had to.

The phone calls she would make to us at the end of each day followed the same pattern for years.

'Hi Ella Bella.'

'Hi Mum. When will you be home?'

'In an hour. Has your brother been dropped off?'

'Yeah. He's upstairs.'

'Good. Can you take the bolognese sauce out of the freezer?'

'Sure. Oh, and can you please get milk on the way home?'

'Okay. Love you.'

I hang up. I set my phone timer and stop thinking about them for a while. I got into that special place where there are no rules, no limits and no brakes. I spin straw into gold – gold that will feed us and pay the bills. Then the buzzer will go off and I'll go home to my kids.

I could pretend the world is different now and your life as a woman is not going to be compromised because of your gender. You're female, but you're also white and first-world and privileged in a thousand ways. Yet even with this powerful scaffolding of advantage around you, there may still be moments when yourself as a woman takes over your *self.*

I can't assure you that this imbalance, this Before and After, this compromise won't continue, but I can ask you to refrain from hiding it.

Do not hide your bleeding, your pain or the movement of yourself from one state to another. Do not sit in a Before or an After. Swing between the two and land somewhere else. Say 'vulva', shake hands with gusto, talk about menopause over dinner. Do not quiet yourself.

Lesson #112: Bleed loudly.

Letter Sixteen

Go far, go wide

Travel makes your eyes bigger. They become pupilled satellite dishes twisting and turning, soaking in every smell and clamour and fear-feeling. To travel is to knock yourself out of routine and be forced to pay attention: the most banal becomes the most fascinating.

Your family has crisscrossed the globe by way of work or war or even simple old pleasure. Travel is what ties many of our stories together. Not so much because it's all we have to tell, but because it's those tales that are most resistant to the fading power of time.

I hope you travel. I hope you get to experience the exultant joy that comes from being somewhere else – far away, the song of another language stirring around you.

In the years that these letters began to take the form of a book, many corners of the world have been locked away from adventure. The spectacular privilege of moaning about travel has been removed from us. We're all now aware of how lucky we were, for all that time, to fly around the world in magical silver tubes. We're all now wondering if we'll ever do it again.

Before I had you, I was scared of flying. I'd drink enough champagne to file down the edges of my fear, close my eyes and focus on the buffeting of the airstreams around the plane.

'If we go down,' I'd mentally chant, a quiet psychic prayer that no-one else could hear:

'If we go down,
please let it be fast enough,
that I won't know,
we didn't make it.'

This is a more depressing (and melodramatic) version of my grandfather's approach. When his parents were visiting in Melbourne in late 1959, they heard that Buzz and Virginia had arranged to send their children off, alone, back to the United States to stay with Virginia's parents. Virginia explains:

> *[His parents] were horrified.*
>
> *'But if their plane crashed, how would you feel?' asked my mother-in-law.*
>
> *'Damn glad I hadn't been on it,' was Jim's reply.*

After you were born, we travelled far and frequently – returning back to your father's birthplace as often as was possible. As you grew from baby to toddler, your awareness of me grew as well. I could not show you I was afraid. I was too busy gripping your hand and saying, brightly:

'Isn't this fun!'

Somehow, along the way, it did become fun.

Lesson #113: Fake it 'til you make it.

I've grown up in a time when air travel is split between Before 2001 and After 2001. You won't know what it was like to travel before fear became a piece of carry-on luggage that we're all expected to bring along with us. Some hold it tighter than others. I remember one flight when you were a baby. We were returning home from the UK, hurtling somewhere between London and Singapore. When, in the muddied gloom of the plane-night when everyone is pretending to sleep and the air is full of stale breath, I heard a commotion. You do not want to hear a commotion on a plane.

There was an ill passenger and the flight attendant was running away down the aisle. You do not want to hear running on a plane.

There was beeping and raised voices, and I kept my eyes squeezed shut hoping you wouldn't wake up, hoping you would stay snuggled in your little air-cot. And then I peeked and spied the thin line on the digital map before me begin to loop like a slow boomerang. The plane was turning. We were folding back on ourselves and I knew the long night was about to get longer. You do not want to see the plane turning around. Luckily, I didn't have to become as involved as Buzz did, flying from Yemen:

> *We got on the plane to go to Djibouti ... It was just a freight type plane with bench seats. It was loaded with Qat, a narcotic leaf they chew in the Arab states. So we got onto this very old DC3. It had cracks around the door. Two Ethiopian pilots. I felt pretty safe. We would be flying over the desert and could make an emergency landing anywhere. An old man got in with a hibachi type thing. I thought he was just carrying it but he put it down and after we took off he proceeded to build a fire. I went up to the cockpit door and banged on it and brought the co-pilot back. He came and grabbed the man by the neck and hit him a few times. The co-pilot then put out the fire. As we flew along I thought the sun's in the wrong place for where we were going and sure enough, when he hit the Red Sea the pilot made a ninety degree turn and headed to Djibouti. When we got on the ground I asked him why he did that and he said he was day dreaming. He said as soon as he saw the Red Sea he knew what he'd done.*

We spent nearly thirty hours on that plane, between London and Singapore and back to Dubai before landing in Melbourne. It was my pre-baby nightmare come true. Yet I had all my energy focused on entertaining you, jiggling you up and down in the blue light of the kitchenette, besocked-feet cold on the steel floor. And when we arrived home, I took an internal flight manifest. The passenger was okay. You were okay. I was okay.

I still don't love planes.

Regardless, I'm taking you on a little trip. Fear of flying be damned: in this letter you and I are going travelling. Much like Jim, you will not need a passport – not this time, anyway. But I mean it. We are going travelling – you and I, right now! Yes, even in the middle of this pandemic.

In this plane, that you and I are travelling on, there will be no boomerang U-turns, no open fires and no stale mouth-air. This time I won't be faking the happiness, I am much better on planes now. I think we should fly on something like the Super Constellation that Buzz and Virginia took to Australia in 1958. I'm sure it's a bit noisier than the modern planes, but the bunk beds and downstairs bar should make up for it.

> *[The] Pan Am Super Constellation droned across the Pacific. The bunks ... were welcome. The long trip was made easier by the bar downstairs in the belly of the plane, which served as a playroom some of the time with colouring books for the children.*

Our first stop is France. My great-grampa, Jim, loved France.

His letters back to Kay from the Great War sing of a country that I've certainly never experienced. I'm not sure anyone could; not now. Not only would one have to travel to France, but one would have to travel to 1918. And would need to be wearing the rosy-hued glasses of a 24-year-old man in Europe for the first time, full of love, and sitting with the knowledge that he may not come home:

> *As for me here – La-la! – Pouf! as the natives would say. I'm getting along fine. I'm having a chance to see French peasant life*

as I could never hope to in any other way. C'est an experience and, as I have said before, a life is a series of experiences – so this is some life …

There is nothing in existence to rival the peace and content that spreads itself over a French village at twilight. The cows come plodding home and the sheep, herded into separate lots by intelligent mongrels, trot in a restless mass down the street. On every doorstep sit three or four doughboys trying to overcome the common barriers of speech and earnestly assuring the wondering villagers that a combination of [Lingo, Patois and Profanity] is pure French. All this through my window – which after all is a good window with lace curtains for screens and grey stones for a setting and geraniums for adornment.

Jim had to redact his location from his letters to Kay, but later, long after the war had finished, he revealed he had been training up in the Haute-Marne country. Jim loved France. So did Virginia. Four decades after the training was over (and the fighting the training was for), Jim's daughter Virginia and her husband found themselves in another quaint French village, only 200 kilometres west from where her father had billeted:

Roughly halfway between Geneva and Paris we came into Auxerre. A town which to our eyes, seemed so typically French as to be irresistible. On the highest point was the cathedral with buttresses flying, stained glass glowing. Narrow cobbled streets tumbled down from there, losing themselves in a labyrinth of half-timbered buildings, some of them four storeys tall and overhanging the lanes to an alarming degree. But nowhere could we find a place to spend the night. Finally we found an establishment which welcomed us after hearing Buzz's impassioned plea on behalf of his pregnant wife.

'Mais oui, mais oui!' exclaimed the proprietor, a plump madame in black. We heard running feet and whispers before Madame showed us up to our lovely room.

'Madame,' Buzz said to me after she had left us. 'That's what she is, I'll bet. This is a brothel, I can feel it!'

I refrained from asking just how he knew the feel of a brothel. I was too grateful for a night's sleep in the clean, comfortable bed.

Lesson #114: When travelling, it's sometimes best to refrain from asking questions.

My journeying through France was a lot less extensive and a lot more sedate than Grama's or Great-Grampa's respective visits. I've not spent any time out of Paris, and the time I've spent in that city has been short. It was a weekend trip, through some requirements of my working holiday visa – this was a time when the bureaucrats of the world encouraged you to cross borders, rather than the opposite. I've spoken to you about the food we ate in that city, but not much else. Tom and I stayed in a hotel so small that our bags didn't fit into the elevator at the same time as we did.

So for you and me, our time in France will be focused more on the countryside than the city. It's where we have more stories to reread, and more adventures to repeat. Jim spent more time in France post-Armistice than he did during his months of fighting.

It was after he'd been discharged from the officers' hospital in London that he ended up back in Paris – however, he was there without any special orders, which isn't advised when you're an officer in the United States Army:

I was taken before the chief judge of the military police. And I looked up at him, he looked down at me, and who do you suppose he was? He had been the captain of the cavalry unit I had served with [five years earlier] on the border of Texas, in Eagle Pass. Talk about the odds and the luck being with you!

He said, 'I know what I'll do, Jim. I'll give you an order enabling you to travel all over France looking for your lost baggage.'

> *So he gave me such an order, and I ended up having quite a time, quite a tour for myself of France.*

My love, Jim had not lost any luggage at all.

On our trip, this magical tour, you and I will travel the French countryside like your great-great-grandfather did. We'll eat ripe yellow plums followed by juicy roast chicken, and drink champagne. (I am assuming, in this trip, you are Of Age.)

*

> *Prunes [sic] are ripe here and Madame brings us in a plate of different kinds every day. Blue ones, and big yellow ones, and little yellow ones, and all of them very good. We count the old lady in on our champagne parties every once in a while and she contributes with a brand of eau-de-vie that has to be mixed with five parts water to keep it from bursting into flame. Today she has promised to make us some prune tarts for 'after supper'. Some old lady is Madame.*

During this visit, however, it will help if one of us speaks the language. Do you speak French, *ma chérie*? You don't now, of course, but maybe by the time you read this letter and we are ready to fly around the world together, you will. I hope so, because I certainly don't. Throughout my schooling, I attempted to learn eleven languages and never learned more than 'Hello' in a few of them. This is outrageous.

I'm not sure how much French Jim spoke, but he certainly forgave those Frenchpersons he met who did not speak English back to him:

> *In the French city of [—] we met Jane. She was all that my fevered imagination had suggested that a cafe girl ought to be and she spoke English with an accent novelists speak of as 'charmingly*

broken' meaning that you couldn't understand her. She also had the English faculty of charging three times what her champagne was worth, so that before we got through we were all charmingly broke.

On the Saturday of our Parisian weekend Tom and I walked like people do when they're in a city they don't belong to. After three years of French lessons at school I was dismayed to realise – in the middle of Paris – I knew three words. At a word per year, that's not 'charmingly broken', it's 'bloody embarrassing'.

Not speaking the language made me feel so impotent; so frustrated. I implored with my eyes, embarrassed, willing them to understand me. But Tom spoke French, so I was saved.

All my travels have made me realise what a currency the spoken word is. Hearing the handsome man with blue eyes beside me speak French made me realise it was as much a currency for me as it was for him.

Wouldn't be a bad plan for me to go to Italy, would it? Maybe I could learn a new language so that there'd be a few more pet names for me to think of you by. Two or three more languages and I could come somewhere near the number of pet names you deserve, Lady o' mine.

Lesson #115: Learn a language.

Once we have traversed France we will move on to Italy. This is where my heart sings more loudly than anywhere else. My first experience of Italy was Puglia. All I knew was that Tom and I were heading for the 'heel of the boot'. It was July and we left an oppressive, humid London for the sharp heat of Southern Italy. We picked up our car at Bari Airport and I watched Tom keep us alive on the Italian *superstrada* while I white-knuckled along beside him.

We eventually found our way through the bone-dry olive groves and weekend-silent towns to arrive at the small collection of white *trulli* in which we were staying. It was a patchwork of flowerpots, mismatched furniture, geraniums and heavy bougainvillea. A gaggle of puppies with spaghetti limbs lolloped over our toes. Our host removed himself from the chickens he was tending to show us our cool, dark *trullo.* We drank too much Italian white on our little terrace under the fig tree, avoiding its overripe missiles that started to drop as the sun went down. We unwound from the tension of living and working in a big city. We cooked pasta with tiny tomatoes.

We will go there, you and I, and we will eat tiny tomatoes, followed by wind-felled figs.

*

The heat in Southern Italy is dry and brutal. In 2005 it was a shock to this Australian whose blood had been chilled by English winters. Luckily, the sea was not far from where we stayed. When your father and I visited, we set off for a locals-only beach in Torre Guaceto, eventually – after many wrong turns and long roads – finding a rugged little cove with aquamarine water and chocolate-brown Italians. Just like your father and I did, you and I will sit in the glaring sun and swim through the blue-glass Adriatic when it becomes too hot. All the time we'll keep an eye on the multiple Italian generations crowding under umbrellas, eating, gesticulating, sunbaking. Together we will wonder, how can so many people be such a smooth, uniform bronze? That night we will fall asleep in the same way I did all those years ago – with hair full of Italian seawater and ears full of the sound of frisky puppies.

We've already discussed the importance of the sea, but when travelling it's all the more crucial – if you can, swim at the local beach. A beach off the tourist track is much like a local supermarket: you will see and know more about where you're travelling than in most other places.

Lesson #116: Travel makes even the ordinary, worthy.

We needn't stop after France and Italy, my girl. Let's make it just the beginning. I may rest a little but you can travel as far as your ancestors. You have it in your blood.

In the 1960s, Buzz and Virginia took a tour around the world in between overseas postings. Their itinerary 'sent shivers up Virginia's spine', and envy down my own: Singapore, Bangkok, Hong Kong, Delhi, Cairo, Athens, Rome, Naples, Geneva, Paris, London, New York.

And Kay's matter-of-fact descriptions of her own travels put mine, again, to shame. In 1974 she wrote of a dizzying array of destinations:

> *During the past twenty years we have spent many of our vacations travelling, inspired partly by the fact that Jim and Virginia have lived overseas. In 1952 we went to Mexico, and in 1955 we made our first trip to Europe. In 1959 we went around the world and in 1964 we visited Jim and Virginia in Kenya and included in that trip stops in Egypt, Greece, Spain and Portugal …*

By 1967, Buzz and Virginia were settled back into that 'comfortable, suburban life' in the country they had left nearly a decade before. They and their three children had moved from Ghana to a pretty white house with a red roof on Saugatuck Shores. Living on an island off Westport, Connecticut, meant they were 60 metres from Long Island Sound. But returning 'home' to the United States was not as simple as they'd hoped. Buzz's experience of an airlock inside a New York office meant it was a particularly grey time for him.

My grandparents travelled further and for longer than they both imagined for themselves or their family. But now they were settled back in America, Buzz was taking more trips without his wife and children. He would bring back rich gifts from places once frequented by them both. Grama remembers,

> *When Buzz returned from Paris in December of 1968 he brought me a loaf of bread, a lump of cheese and a rosebud.*

Yet it wasn't just gifts he bore, but the knowledge shared with his wife that some of the places they had left might be ready for their return:

> *These working holidays relieved the monotony of New York but a visit to Melbourne made it somehow more difficult. He wrote [to me] 'It's painful to come back on just a short visit. This place and the people are even better than we remembered them.'*

With their own exotic travels around the globe, and Virginia's parents' similar itineraries, it might be difficult to understand why Buzz and Virginia ended up living in a relatively small city at the bottom of the world.

As with most important decisions around travel, it may have been influenced by the people, more than the place. Virginia's father, Jim, had his own agreeable experience with Australians in his war – and a theory about why it was so:

> *I sometimes think about when we brigaded with the ANZACs: the Australian-New Zealand Army Corps. These two groups of men got along wonderfully; they were buddies, you know. My men couldn't understand the lingo that the Australians were speaking most of the time, but their backgrounds were the same. Same gold rushes, the same one generation of settlers behind them, same in the way of being cattlemen and sheepmen, and they got along.*

Whereas, differently, when we were brigaded with the British we did more fighting with them than we did with the Germans. Now, the Australians today are naturally friendly to … a man from the western part of the United States. But not to a New Englander. So I have developed a theory that an outgoing willingness to be friendly to a stranger is in inverse ratio to the number of generations the frontier is behind you.

Travel is wonderful because it paves a way from the place you left to the place you return to. Sometimes this road takes you far over the horizon. Sometimes it takes you home. Buzz and Virginia's first time in Melbourne had resonated in a way they did not expect, and in 1969 they had decided it was the city to which they would return.

We looked around the Connecticut house, at the mementoes of our former life. The boomerangs, carvings, gold weights, Kente cloth and masks we'd brought from far away which made the island feel like home. An eclectic decor within which we found solace in our memories. These souvenirs comforted us at first then began to rankle as we grew to realise there was little chance of further overseas postings.

Virginia later wrote of the moment when their next destination was sealed as their final one. Buzz had flown from New York to Melbourne for an interview in a role that would bring all the family back to Australia. She explains the moment it was confirmed for her husband:

[The interviews] went well. [They] liked Jim, liked what he'd done in the past and were eager to have him work for them in the future.

Jim cabled me 'Ndio, ndio, ndio!' (Swahili for 'Yes, yes, yes!') and the die was cast.

And as Buzz said:

> *Then off to Melbourne. This was 1969 [and] it was the best thing we ever did.*

My girl, travel is a gift and a privilege and if you ever have the opportunity, you must run very fast at it. Your family is made up of travellers, but that is not why you should join us. Do it for yourself. Travel will show you what is different and what is the same. Travel will teach you what is important and what isn't.

Lesson #117: Travel to find your home.

Letter Seventeen

Turning on myself

I have been lying to you since you were born. As I write these letters, I'm still lying to you.

Having a baby is to have a little fleshy god descend from above, and land into your world. Babies watch everything, but see little: they are omnipotent in all but understanding. As a new mother I lived my whole life with you in the audience – nothing was off limits. I sat on the toilet with you suckling at my breast, I vomited with your toddler hand gripping my back, I changed my tampon in cramped shopping-centre toilet stalls while you watched from close quarters. Does this disgust you? It shouldn't. It didn't then.

Being a mother of a very young child is to become completely exposed, because there is nowhere else for you (or them) to go. A child's all-seeingness removes any room for vanity, decorum or modesty.

Yet putting the brutal intimacy of bodily fluids aside, in those early days, it was easy to deceive you.

Now, you are older. We rarely share a bathroom stall. But you see more, and you hear everything. Your eyes narrow and lips purse, and I wonder at what age you'll realise the extent of my deception. Or if you already have?

I have lied to others. Lovers, friends, strangers. But the lies have changed. I used to protect my truth of how hungry I was. Now I protect my truth of how much I still desire to be hungry. And how I equate it all with being beautiful.

I often wonder if it's just me. If every other mother around me is as confident and accepting as they project they are. As I've been told *I* should be. As I pretend I am to you.

Sometimes the truth seeps out and I glimpse someone who is living the same lie as I am.

Gastro is going around: 'Oh, give it to me, I could lose a few kilos.'

School pick-up reveals a suddenly smaller mother: 'She's on her son's ADHD meds.'

I am diagnosed with cancer: 'At least I'll be thin now.' (Spoiler: I wasn't.)

Lesson #118: Don't weigh yourself. Don't diet.
Don't hate your body. I will beg: <u>please</u>.

I wanted to make sure I wasn't alone, so I asked other women – some friends, most strangers – if they felt the same. And they did. The overwhelming, depressing majority of us are still trying to change the way our bodies look. When we were young, we lied about how much food we avoided, how hungry we were, how much we vomited it up.

Now we are older, we lie that we no longer care: that we embrace our 'tiger stripes' and 'mother bellies' and 'glorious wobbly bits'. We don't diet: we cleanse. We don't count calories: we count affirmations. We don't starve: we fast. We accept our flaws and never say 'fat' – and we lie, and lie, and lie.

We just keep lying.

Hardwiring is a bitch.

In my reality, the ultimate victory has always been to be thin, to be strong, to be fit, but to never acknowledge any of it. To not show any attempt at achieving or maintaining. In the internal world I inhabit, it's not enough to be the 'perfect' size and shape – you must do so without any effort. You must fall into perfection by accident. Like tripping into a puddle of glowing skin and angular cheekbones.

As I write this letter I am embarking on yet another diet. No-one knows. Just my husband and my mother. I'm ashamed to have gained and I'm more ashamed to be trying to lose it. Where is the ethereal state of self-acceptance that exists outside this cycle of punishment? Is it a meditation I haven't discovered yet? Or is the ADHD rumour not actually a rumour?

I'm sorry, my love. I wish this could be an affirmative, strong, positive tale that you hold close to yourself and smile at. At this, I have failed. I am the alcoholic writing my story of addiction while still drunk. Yet it doesn't feel so extreme because everyone I know is quietly trying to change their body as well. We are all drunk and we are all pretending to be in recovery.

Lesson #119: Try to forgive me.

I could blame the patriarchy. I could blame the media. I could blame my own family. It's all of them. My generation and the women before me teenaged through angular models and actresses, hip bones sharp and clavicles deep. There is a social media video I saw recently that showed a rapid-fire montage of paparazzi photos from magazines fifteen years ago. Photos I still remember vividly. The clips made me wince. I knew those girls were slim then. Now I think they were ill.

Recently, you and I have been watching 1990s and noughties rom-coms together. They're filled with the shadows of my teens, and an innocence that later films don't hold for me anymore. Regardless, I'm aware of how my nostalgia can cloud things, so I always check their rating and reviews before we dive in. Language, sex, violence – I check and balance all the prospective inappropriateness before we press play. But as we tick more and more films off, I realise that the three pillars of Profanity, Porn and Punching are nothing compared to the systemic and incessant referencing of women's bodies, dieting and 'fatness'. And when the words aren't talking about mass, the actresses' bodies are. The heroes are thin. THIN. Not twenty-first century slim, but angular, angrily, ailingly thin.

Mamma Mia, *Notting Hill*, *How to Lose a Guy in Ten Days*, *Love Actually*, *Clueless*, *Never Been Kissed*, *You've Got Mail*.

Throwaway pieces of dialogue that stick in the throat.

'I don't want people saying, "There goes that famous actor with the big, fat girlfriend".'

'Anyway, I know why he dumped me: I'm too fat!'

'He says no-one's going to fancy a girl with thighs the size of big tree trunks.'

We watched too many before I had the sense to stop watching them at all.

Lesson #120: Try to forgive all of us.

So there are endless layers of indoctrination, public and private. It's something we've all been educated on (but still, somehow, not vaccinated against). So I don't know why I was surprised when I, one woman, realised something with a sinking inevitability. I couldn't rewire my own consciousness in the thirteen months it took for you, my perfect baby, to gain sentient language. However, once you were born I tried very hard to become a poster child for physical forgiveness. I think it worked, for a few years at least.

I banned the 'f' word for as long as I could in this house: not 'fuck', but 'fat'. I would have flinched much more to hear you say the latter than the former. So much so that when you first spied Monty Python's grotesquely obese character Mr Creosote you whispered, all of the age of three, 'That man is very … *large*.'

It's not hard to see that this censorship was much more about me than it was about your sensitivities. Even so, we go on – you get older – and we continue to talk about 'rainbow plates' and 'sometimes foods' and I wonder where the line is blurring between me educating you and you educating me.

Because in some way, and by 'some' I mean – this fucking bullshit – in this fucking bullshit way, it's worse now. Because it's not better. It's just not obvious any more. It's not overt. Now not only are we held to the standards built by the patriarchy and media and fashion and diet culture ... now we're also held to the standard of being positive role models. And being 'wholesome' and 'holistic' and 'balanced'. Social media means I can share to a few thousand people that I am having a bad mental health day but if I tell anyone I am uncomfortable in my skin, or I want my belly to be smaller, then I am not playing by the new rules. And all these shifts would make sense if the inner was reflecting the outer. But it's not. We're still fucked-up inside.

So this is why I've been lying to you. Why when I grab my stomach rolls with a big smile on my face, my internal monologue is hissing: *Ugh, look at it, it's never been this big.* When I jiggle my bum in its big undies, while you laugh: *God, these are bigger than my pregnancy knickers were.* When I eat the last bite of cheesecake you've offered me: 'Mmm yum!' *I am so pathetic – where is my self-control?*

Lesson #121: Have a child so you have to pretend to be brave.

In digging through my past I have been saddened – devastated, really – to read how deep and for how long this cruelty has been sitting with me. At each phase in my life I think I believed I was being subtle. Private diary entries, yes. But public group emails to friends and relatives, outlining my weight gain in numbers? It's harrowing. Humiliating. How did I not question this? How did no-one else? How then, as a mother, did I ever think that something as deeply ingrained in my being could be hidden from something else that has come from that same being, sewn from that same thread?

My first dramatic weight loss was after my first dramatic break-up and I was curious to feel the clothes hanging from my body rather than gripping it. I navigated a life where food was low down on the priority list, behind dancing, booze and falling in love. A journey to London was a trigger and I weighed myself in the Boots pharmacy at Hays Galleria once a week, documenting the 100-gram incremental increases with rising panic.

My years in London have left behind a breadcrumb trail of little scraps of sad poetry. A list of my daily food intake fills corners of every workbook, diary, notepad and calendar. A mangled, coded haiku to control (a tick day) and regret (a cross day): Apple, Ryebread w. beans & Mango, nuts, Ch salad, yo. That's not right. My grade five English teacher would be ashamed. Let's try again.

Apple, then ryebread
and beans. Mango, then nuts and
chook salad, yoghurt.
<fin>

There was a period of years after returning to Melbourne when weight faded into the background and I found an almost-utopia where I was not dieting and miserable. There are still spikes of recalled-remorse, like the time *as a manager* of a team, I created a calendar in which the women I worked with each ticked off a box for days of 'Exercise, Good Food and No Booze'. I printed one off for each woman and pinned them over our desks. I'm so sorry, team.

But in general, at that time, my body was healthy. I liked food. I was not racked with obsession. I achieved this state both pre- and post-pregnancy. A decade of distraction from the guilt. Until cancer, menopause, a pandemic and – ultimately – the bottom of a very deep hole of over-reward, guilt, consumption and Ice Magic.

This is the most shameful letter I will include in this package for you. Because I am revealing to you what I've never said out loud to anybody else: I have golden core memories of moments that shouldn't be remembered, and certainly shouldn't be gilded. I can recall every moment in the past fifteen years when someone has remarked how thin I was. I can tell you exactly where I was (the office kitchen on Ferrars Street, the timber table at number 38, the mirrored wardrobe in Marylebone, the library floor in South Yarra), and what it felt like (a gleeful rush of relief and success at knowing that I was Doing It).

I can tell you that those moments are memorable because of how fleeting they were. A little breath of wind in a still, endless summer of calorie counting, restricting and bingeing. It's never until years later that I look back at photos and realise how perfect I was – on days I thought I wasn't. And every year that passes, the preceding year's photographs develop beauty like I develop hindsight. I see those photographs and wonder why I spent so much time worrying. I see them and still my brain tells me how ugly and fat I am today. Today is the day I have hit rock-bottom. Today I am the most fat. In a year the past-me will be perfect, I guess. But it will be too late. In a year the today-me will be ugly and fat again.

I can tell you that when I have been truly, deeply afraid – whether it's when I have been waiting for my PET scan results, or the MRI results from your own perfect body – I have prayed to whatever god I think will listen and apologised. I've regretted for every moment I've ever wasted on trying to carve my body and my psyche into a different shapes. I've pleaded with those gods that I promise promise promise I will never take my healthy, strong body for granted if only they will let you be well, or let me live.

And then, faster than you can possibly imagine, I go back to hating my body and trying to change it.

I began this letter on the first day of a new diet. You are too aware for me to manage this under your nose without you noticing. But I proceed anyway. I know I am creating a fissure in your consciousness by doing this in front of you. I am so sorry. But I can't stop. I am overweight, my bras are metal corsets digging into my rib cage and I am desperate. I tell myself that if I lose kilograms, I will be lighter and brighter and more positive and you will notice that more than you noticed how I got there. I tell myself; I lie to myself.

You'll also notice this letter is the only one in which my words sit alone. I have not blended any of Jim, or Buzz's, or Virginia's or Kate's, or anyone else's words in here. I want my words to sit here without relief or historical insulation. I imagine the women in my family had their hunger. I know they had their moments of sadness and disgrace. But these words are mine to share, today.

A memory that feels more awful than anything else I've related here, is the moment you pointed at your own perfect body and told me it was wrong. Your cheeks; your belly: you didn't like them. Someone had teased you. Someone had made you feel imperfect. You were sitting in your top bunk and it was way past bedtime and a chill set into the pit of my stomach, like I'd swallowed poison. I said the right words and you went to sleep. As I left your bedroom I felt like Pandora's Box had finally opened – after I'd been kicking at it for five years.

I don't know what will happen as you grow into the danger years of body image. I don't know how to fix all the mess I've spilled across your subconscious. But I do promise you that this letter, if it ever makes it into the light of day – will be my exorcism.

I stand before you, the only hopes I have remain held, one in each hand:

1. Now I have said these words aloud, I am not lying anymore.
2. I have been well before, which means I can be well again.

Lesson #122: Have a child so you will be brave.

Letter Eighteen

Find yourself a coven

Coven

/ˈkʌv(ə)n/ – Noun

1. *A group or meeting of witches.* 2. *A secret or close-knit group of associates.*

This is a letter to tell you about the friends and mothers in my life, and yours, and what I have learned from them all.

I have mothers (plural) and I have friends (plural). Together they form the brethren who have kept me going during the lowest times. They have filled up my tank over and over, often to the point where I can fill up others. This is the village. This is the coven. This is why we surround ourselves with good people. You are welcome to join mine, just as I skirted around my own mother's for a time. But you will also grow your own, of that I'm sure. Because connection is the electrical impulse that inevitably sparks up between two living things, whether you want it or not. And the ensuing friendship can help you survive during the dark days, and grow during the others.

But first:

This is not a letter to tell you how to make friends.

(But, in case you're wondering: ask questions, listen to the answers, keep their secrets, remember what was said the next time you see them, ask more questions, repeat.)

This is not a letter to tell you how to be a mother.

(But, in case you're wondering: birthing a human is not necessary. Just provide unconditional love and the feeling of safety, and you will be a mother).

When your father leaves you at eight years old, your life becomes inherently more female. My mother had a latticework of women around her, bearing the load. Over the thirteen years between my father leaving and my leaving, our house was filled with the steady spirit of strong women. But this energy did not just come from my mother's friends. As I grew older, I was lucky enough to be encircled by a broader group of female forces, many of them mothers. Most of them women. I was born from them and loved by them. And so are you, now.

The first mother

I met my great-grandmother Kay twice, the last time was eight years before her death. It was 1993, and Great-Grama was living in the same Palo Alto house that she and Jim had built from that orchid-adorned property deed some sixty years earlier. Old people can be scary to us young ones, particularly when they sit papery and quiet in a wheelchair, translucent hands revealing thick blue veins. But she was kind, and her eyes were curious. While I wasn't scared, I also wasn't as affected as I should have been. At thirteen, I did not know quite how impressive the woman I was standing beside was. I didn't know, until these letters sent me searching for her words. You, my love, brought me closer to Katherine, and introduced me to the version of her that Jim called Kay. Thank you.

In her brief, deliberate 'Family Record', Kay's journalism background lays out her life story with an understated power. With an efficient turn of phrase, she outlines in five pages what the men around her do in a hundred. Kay was a pioneer in female achievement but you wouldn't know it to read her words. Listen to her:

> *After my father died I went to work for the Long Beach Press and also did volunteer publicity for the Red Cross. After the Armistice we were transferred to a Motor Transport Unit … We arrived in Texas on May 5th and spent the next four months working hard, trying unsuccessfully to keep cool and battling various forms of insect life: weevils in the flour, cockroaches in the sink and a scorpion in the laundry bag.*
>
> *[After the war] there was a job open in the circulation department of the Press and I went to work there at $15.00 a week. Before long I was given a raise.*

Kay was twenty-two and women were still two years away from being allowed to vote.

I had to try harder to find these accounts than I tried for anyone else's in this family. Kay was understated, even in death. Her obituary was written by her middle child, the son who helped locate her 'Family Record' for me, in 2021.

> *She was quite an outdoors woman for her generation, a good shot with a shotgun and an excellent trout fisher… She and my father were among the early devotees of mule pack trips in the High Sierra in the 1920s and '30s.*

Kay was, by all accounts, an 'exacting' woman, but with a sparkle of knowing in her eye. It makes me sad that there isn't the same volume of Kay's own words to draw on as there are others, to stir through these letters to you. But then, I have many other women who arrived in her wake, to tell us more. Her daughter Virginia related this anecdote, which may tell us more about her mother than much else:

> *[Mother's dress] was a purple crepe gown with spaghetti straps, skintight until it flared out from thigh to ankle. When my*

daughter found it hanging forgotten in a closet years later, she begged her grandmother's permission to try it on. Then wailed, 'But Grama, it shows my underwear!'

'I wore no pants or bra with that dress' was her calm reply.

The grandmother

Not Grandma, *Grama*. Virginia has never been rosewater and thick stockings. No, you can't be, with a face like Ava Gardner, jet-black hair and legs that rocked short-shorts way past the age the rest of us dared to. In these stories, Virginia is my Grama. But she is also Mum's Mum, your 'GG', Buzz's 'Quig', and she was her father's 'Half Pint'. No matter what name tag she happens to be wearing, Grama has maintained a slightly intimidating glamour through all stages. Now in her mid-nineties, she drinks champagne and flirts with the blokes at her aged-care home. Due to Covid, I see her less than ever before, but we speak often. When I was having cancer treatment she began sending me snippets of memories accompanied by photographs. Every day, a different email; brief, magical and just begging for more explanation. With her pith and one-liners, she taught me more than any writer's group could. As I and the rest of the world grew dusty in lockdown, I started to share 'Questions for Grama' (and her responses) to the internet. These exchanges were some of my favourite moments of the pandemic. In these emails were some of the seeds from which these letters sprouted.

Q. What hors d'oeuvres would you serve at a party?
A. I come from a generation that made fiddly hors d'oeuvres. Stuffed olives wrapped in bacon and browned under the griller. Smoked oysters on little toast rounds. My mother used to pride herself on her Bovril crisps.

Q. Did your father only have one martini?
A. Mother had just one in her special little glass, Daddy had at least two saying there was a dividend, the last drop from the martini jug. A maths teacher once asked if anyone knew what a dividend was and I answered 'the last martini in the jug'. Someone once gave Daddy a handblown crystal teapot to mix/ serve his martinis in/from. I knit him a tea cosy to fit.
I'd had several the night I agreed to go to Australia.

Q. What was your most favourite outfit and why?
A. A dress I wore in the forties. Dropped waist, olive green with wide salmon pink horizontal stripes. Because I KNEW I was beautiful. As I am now!

Q. If you could list your tips for a long marriage, what would they be?
A. I know it sounds ridiculous but Buzz and I never argued. And that's not just because one tends to put the dear departed on a pedestal, we really didn't. Good sex is important and adapting that to one's age and health is of prime importance. Another tip would be don't try to have deep and meaningful discussions about contentious issues. Things shrink in importance by morning. And we were in love. And came from a long line of couples in love.

I have told you that, from Grama, I have learned that we were a 'family who thought we were important enough to write it all down'. But in asking her questions, I have learned so much more.

My mother

The one who fed and rocked and wiped and carried me. I stood in front of a room of loved ones at her sixtieth birthday and thanked her for her 'pure, raging, batshit bonkers insanity'. Which is true: your Gaga is not just that in name. Any child of an artist could say the same. When I was growing up, Mum was the kind of mother the other kids wanted, because she drew their portraits on paper napkins with a brilliant fluidity that was still beautiful enough for their mothers to hang, framed, in the living room. Because she received a sweaty-cheeked kiss from Jim Morrison at Staples High in 1967. Because after thirty years in advertising she decided to become a cartoonist for *The New Yorker.* And then she did.

Because she asks questions like, 'Are you happy in your heart?'

What the other kids did not see was the slog, the fear, and the jaw-set determination to Just. Keep. Going. When life wasn't playing fair. The thing about Mum, is she's never made a decision (and she's had to make some doozies) about her career, love or family that I haven't respected. Her integrity has always given me something to aim for, and I hope – my darling – this is a strength that you take and hold – from her; from me; I don't mind. The biggest lesson here is one she's demonstrating today. She and I are true friends, and it's because I love you so much that I'm willing to share her with you.

Just as Grama said to me last week, 'I'm really looking forward to seeing your mum tomorrow. She's one of my best friends but I'm willing to share her with you.'

The stepmother

This is a tricky one, isn't it? This woman, who was so different from my own mother, but helped me grow in so many similar ways. She was much younger than I am now when she met the two kids who came attached to the bloke she'd fallen in love with. She and Dad were living in a flat on St Kilda Road and on my brother and my inaugural weekend visit we made chocolate cake covered with Peppermint Crisp. It was my first experience in diverging lives run in parallel: two houses, two mothers, two chocolate cake recipes. Dad had left his first family for her and because of this, nothing about our relationship came with ease.

Yet three decades and another marriage away, we have love that is welded by understanding. She gave me advice, she gave me love and, along with my father, she gave me one of the greatest gifts: from their marriage came sisters who filled a space I didn't know was empty.

The mother-in-law

The woman who loved my husband first. She met me, just a baby at twenty-two. I was full of vim and vigour but empty of any clue about what life would hold. I remember nervously choosing my outfit for our first meal together: a full, 1950s-style skirt, pale pink and brown stripes, hoping to seem a respectable choice for their son. It didn't last long, as polite inquiry over Sunday lunch unravelled marriages, divorces, steps, overseas journeys and all the other complications that made me such a messy choice for her son. Yet she was, and has always remained, gracious and graceful. She also taught me that a married couple could be still be happy after forty-odd years, something I always worried was just a myth. When Tom moved 19,000 kilometres away from her heart, she just grew her love and sent it further. Since having my own child, this is a sacrifice that I comprehend in an entirely brighter light.

So here we all are. We sound like a serious bunch, but there's a surprising amount of laughter (and cheek, it has to be said). I will always welcome the noise of these women standing together, either in reality or just in my Inner Monologue.

While we all stand together, you'll notice that we make sure there is space left for one other woman. Let's call her 'the Other Mother'. We welcome this woman into our circle, shuffling over to accommodate, her shoulders rubbing on ours. It's important for me to acknowledge her here today. Because I have been this woman. Darling, you may be, one day. The Other Mother has held a baby in her arms, or in her belly, or in her thoughts. She has sat in waiting rooms, in pathology centres, in hospital recovery lounges, and now she sits with us. She has taken her medicine and swilled her herbs and said her silent prayers over and over. While she didn't get the child she wanted, the child who could call her 'Mama', that name still sits in her heart.

We make a space for her in this circle, for what some of us have lost, and what some of us never had. She's welcome for the wisdom and the love she brings.

*

Look at these women! They are forever jostling, teasing, bossing and loving. These are the voices in the gallery that coached me to be a mother myself. You have me, but you also have all of these mothers. A coven that keeps growing.

There's a photograph from my twenty-first birthday. There are women, perfectly lined up in profile so you can see each face. My mother, then her four closest friends. All of them have the same turned, happy look. They are watching me make a speech with an expression that I now recognise as pride and relief and champagne. Years later I would arrive home after midnight and find some of the same seated around the kitchen table, golden with guttering candlelight and saffron risotto, ready for my stories from the evening. They delighted in my successes and were wounded by my tragedies. They were the first to show me what a friendship should be.

Lesson #123: Gather as many mothers as you can muster.

*

My own candlelit brethren are spread much wider than a dinner table. The core began with three girls: two Cs and me. Three girls living within one small suburb, attending the same school. Tied together by the fact that when we met we were the only few whose parents were divorced, who went home on the 'wrong' tram every day.

Jesus. I feel like I'm writing a pastiche of a Liane Moriarty book.

The rest of the school headed east into the leafy suburbs, we took the other tram south, where there were still milk bars and pubs on our street corners. It's laughable now, to think of where we grew up as 'the wrong side of the tracks'. But in 1991 my birthday party was still considered too far away for some of the other-suburb girls.

The three of us have had the rare privilege to meet one another in childhood yet love one another into adulthood. After school, we skipped together into the next, heady phase. Moving in a way, I was already aware, that was special. My mother, who had spent a disjointed childhood making and remaking friends across a dozen schools and countries, had to wait much longer until she and her friends could move the same way.

It was in 1977, with steam blanketing the surface of a sun-warmed swimming pool in California, when 24-year-old Kate swam beneath the dry desert air with people she would go on to call lifelong friends.

> *I can't bear to think it will all end tomorrow. This special place, this freedom, is a revelation to me. I feel young and strong and full of new wisdom. Nothing else could be this glorious.*
>
> *Who knew life could be like this? Is it the same with everyone? No wonder people fight so hard to live. Until now I assumed life was a challenge to be met.*
>
> *'Come on!' I tread water and look at my new friends. New … but already closer to my heart than the friends I had back home. I have found my kind. I belong here.*

As I grew, my group widened but remained intact. Our gang, grazing in the suburb gently bordered by the Park, the Pub, the Cafe and the Tram Line. A Garden of Eden that held us close, safe and without responsibility. Within those borders we could go and do as we pleased. In those just-out-of-school days, we were safer than we realised, and certainly safer than we would be for a long time to come.

I spent more time out in my suburb at night than I ever had before. I'd gone from listening to hot evenings through my flywire to making the sounds I'd heard. But it was the quiet nights that felt most special. Whenever I walked after midnight it was muted, green and lush. The footpaths of our patch were lined with leaves that smelt of maple syrup, and the hushed magic of knowing anything was possible.

There was a year when a tight dozen of us played board games and drank red wine and talked shit for nights and nights. I would wander down to the pub alone in the knowledge that there would always be someone there knowing my name. Like *Cheers*, but with Bettina Liano jeans and rollies. We ate crinkle cut chips with mushroom gravy. We danced at lock-ins. We flirted. God, could we flirt.

We would flirt with anyone who was in the tractor beam of our enthusiastic glee at just how gorgeous we were becoming. We flirted with men, women, old and young. We flirted with ideas and jobs and sometimes (but not really) danger. What a magic year.

Lesson #124: Nostalgia isn't a dirty word.

One of the most wonderful things about growing older is the new friendships you make. As you move through the chapters of study and work and parenthood, and other life estuaries, you'll collect acquaintances. Your dinner table will heave with friends and others. Most will eventually depart. A friendship that fades in, and fades away, is normal. Sometimes there are those who need to be surrendered.

'But Mum, how do I know which friends to leave behind?' you ask. That's easy. If you leave from time spent together feeling depleted rather than energised, that friendship is not serving you. And, I'm afraid, that is what some relationships are. Interactions that take parts of you away, rather than building you up.

Lesson #125: If a friendship is no longer serving you, you are allowed to let it go.

Back to the Coven. With periphery departed, the most precious will remain. The ones who mother, who need mothering, who don't need anything at all. But all of them with the right energy for *you*. These are the ones to treasure. Lean across the table, ask after their heart, tell them all the reasons why you're happy they are with you.

Lesson #126: Tell your friends why you love them. They mightn't know how to love themselves.

I've been lucky enough to have wonderful company seated at my table. A friend from long ago who has held me, and been held, through children, marriages and a lot of faxes. Brave, funny, strong women I've met through work, who have ended up being bones in my own body strengthening me during the hardest of times. Mothers of your friends, who have seen me at my worst and not run away. Neighbours in life as well as proximity. Women I've shared coffee with, shared baby clothes with, shared exercise mats with. If you were to arrive home after midnight, dear heart, you would find us all. Glowing and ready for your stories.

There are two chairs that are often empty. My original two friends. The three of us have been apart for a long time. Over a decade ago, we three left our safely fenced border separately: our lines of travel crossed over but always parted again. We needed our own adventures. We all fell in and out of love. We had babies, we had affairs, we experienced the unimaginable grief of death and single motherhood and illness and loss. We left. They left. I stayed. We found happiness. We had jagged slumps of loneliness. We became lined with age and bedsheets. Our children don't know each other and how our lives are so comically different. One day they will meet and realise how much we love one another. They'll realise that underneath it all, we're still sort of the same.

We've moved from Liane Moriarty to Alison Lester.

Celia rides horses. Charlotte lives in a jungle. Ella wears red lipstick.

Letter Nineteen

Touch

Three squeezes: 'I. Love. You.'

Four squeezes in return: 'I. Love. You. Too.'

Your Gaga started this with me. Maybe Virginia began it with her. My mother and I have held hands across roads, in theatres, on aeroplanes. A secret message between our palms. Then with you, your little hand in mine – we began again. Three squeezes and then four. 'I. Love. You. Too.'

Often, the moments when you need to hear those words the most, are the moments when speaking is just too hard. But it doesn't matter, because we have the power of this Morse code of flesh and love.

My niece, your cousin, was born the week I began this letter. 'Niece', 'cousin' … the first relative of either name for you and me both, and the first newborn in your immediate circle.

You are transfixed by her tiny pink everything.

I am sitting, happily and curiously, with a new sensation: utter love for a baby that is not my own. It helps that I love both her parents just as fiercely. I watched her fingers yesterday, moving like the anemones Gaga and I have talked about. She is so young that her hands are still papery and wrinkled, an origami of newness slowly unfolding from her wet cradle. A photo of Mum's hands holding her new granddaughter's revealed something else. Mum/Gaga/Kate has the hands of a grandmother. An old lady.

Two papery hands, one gripping the finger of another.

'I. Love. You.'

'I. Love. You. Too.'

Assuming I did not die instantly, I hope that someone was holding my hand at the end. It may have been you. If I have stopped tasting, or smelling, at least I will have been able to feel another hand in mine.

What else would you run your fingers along, if it were the last time those tips could graze another texture? Taste, sound and smell are easy to recollect and easier to mourn for. Touch is different. Maybe in correlation with the thousands of nerve endings meticulously threaded through our fingertips, touch is a sense that is exacting and precise. It doesn't seem to conjure up the dreamy memories which many of these letters are fogged with. Which is counterintuitive, because touch is the most passionate of the senses. The most intimate. The most craved.

I know your father's scalp as well as my own, I've run my fingers through his curls so often. Not just his hair – his scalp. I am a phrenologist with the intimate knowledge of one single human's form. But I am learned in more than his scalp. I know the touch of the warm pulse of his neck. The rougher back of his hand and the softer palm. The organic safety of his sleeping form hooked next to me, with a place between his arm and his heart for me to curl into. When we are apart for longer times, it's this form that I miss. No wonder separation, whether by death or distance or despair; no wonder it can feel so bloody.

After seventeen years of sleeping together, Tom and I have knitted skin.

*

When Jim was nearing the end of his time in Europe, the fervour in his letters is turned up. Enough generations have passed that reading the white-hot desire of this young man (who happens to be my great-grandfather) does not feel icky. It feels deeply, keenly organic:

> *And you say you're a vain girl. Wow! I've known others who could put you in the shade in that one attribute. I don't blame you for being proud of your hair – I'm proud of it, too. Oh, Girl, when you write things like that – the little human touch of you in them makes me hungry for the sight of you.*

The closer his letters get to the end of his war, the more frequently Jim mentions touching his Kay. If this is the passion he commits to paper, then I can't imagine the flaming ball of desire that flew into Washington that day in 1919.

> *[I] don't think of your hair, nor the blackness of its shadows round me – I don't think of the curve of your neck where it slants into your shoulder – nor of the wonderful tomorrows in the distance back of your eyes – nor yet of your fingers on my hair.*
>
> *I think, rather, of all these things when I think of you – and I think most of the pulsing youth that is part of you – and Girl, Girl – I am hungry to be with you again.*

Lesson #127: Absence makes the heart burn, burn white-hot.

When I had finally left London for good, I didn't know if I was leaving your father for good, too. I hoped not. At the departure gates he gifted me a box that contained one of his most treasured items – Ted. The small, misshapen woollen bear had been knitted and repaired so often, his original form was now oversewn a hundred times. I knew how special this object was to Tom and what it meant: a complicit hostage scenario. If I was taking His Ted, then Tom would follow.

For five months I slept with Ted's soft, yet scratchy form in one hand and my solid, twentieth-century phone in the other. Nokia battery burning hot at my fingers, Ted watching in the light of the glowing screen: together, they tethered me back to my love, a hemisphere away. He felt very far off on the other side of the world, but we never considered each other untouchable.

No matter how many leaps technology can make, digital faces and video-hugs can't replace the satiating power of real touch. The pandemic stopped us making physical contact with the people we love who are far away, and made the people who weren't very far seem just as distant. Now we are opening back up, to touch someone seems more reverential an activity than ever before. Kissing, hugging, squeezing hands – these gestures are now graced with the veneration of any previously forbidden activity.

Before travel was locked-away, we would zoom down freeways and hurtle through the sky with a hop and a skip. Our little family would fly through nine time zones to get back to your Mimi and Papa, Tom's parents, without much more thought than visiting Grama down the coast. Now we plan to do the same trip with intent and wonder, and hope. Because at the other end will be people we have not held for a long time.

Lesson #128: Cherish what you can touch, while you can.

Tom's family live in a magical part of England where fairies flit through woods and Christopher Robin played Pooh Sticks over brooks filled with rain.

We have spent some Waugh-worthy summers in East Sussex. I've told you about the dragonflies and sunbeams. But it's also a time when bumblebees drone like heavy blimps through nodding roses and the gin and tonics are always ready at five. One summer's afternoon, when you were about two, we were walking through the neighbour's garden. You were of the age where walks around ponds were more than enough to entertain you, and this pond in particular worked wonders as it had a) a bridge, and b) a healthy population of carp. We had a small butterfly net with us, and your Papa was helping you scoop up fishies to say hello. I can still see you, chubby feet strapped into sturdy sandals, nappy making your bottom square. Before any of us could react, you grabbed one of the fish from the net and planted a kiss on its gaping mouth. The video from my phone has me laughing in shock as you throw it back into the brown water. A proper little Rex Hunt. Do you remember the slime of the brown fish, and why you kissed it?

Those magical summers, that magical time, when those who are no longer, were still with us. Why, I would have kissed a hundred fish: there was that much joy to be shared.

As children we *feel* more than we ever do again. We touch the world when we are closer to the ground and the things that it contains. It's an acquaintance that can be lost. But you and I, girl – right now, we're down in the sand scraping the grains until we hit water. We're climbing trees with fingernails picking at sap. Our knees graze bitumen and bleed into the dirt. We're kissing fish before they flip-slip back into the water.

Lesson #129: Keep holding your hands out.

When Buzz was a boy of nine, he was still living in Fayetteville, Arkansas; not yet having moved out to California with his adoptive parents. He had a friend, Jack, with wiser and older years of twelve. Being kids, they explored the mountainous country behind his house with a recklessness that didn't seem reckless until many years later. Buzz said:

We found a cave system, [we] obtained candles and balls of string [and we stuck the candles to the] wooden paddles. Not telling our folks anything we set off to explore the caves. We let the string out as we went in so we could find our way out if we got lost or the candles burned out. I shudder to think of the small openings we crawled through and the bottomless holes we scrambled over.

Lesson #130: Do not go into that cave.

I shudder, too. I shudder at all the near-misses every child in this story has had, and how they do not become near-misses until something terrible happens to someone else. At the time, it's just childhood. Although as far as I know your childhood has not included scrambling through unmapped caves with only string and candles to guide you.

We eventually found a large cavern. The walls and ceiling were covered in bats. We captured eleven bats and took them home to my basement. We had them in a box but somehow they got out. We had to tell my mother. She said, 'How many you say – eleven? I want to see eleven bats dead or alive by this afternoon.'

Jack and I got two bath towels and thoroughly wet them. One of us with a stick would poke around the rafters in the basement. When one [bat] would fly out, the other guy would hit it with the wet towel.

We got all eleven out alive.

You have managed to avoid introducing wildlife to our home in the nine years you've existed. Thankfully. My brother – your uncle – on the other hand, tended to touch, hold and bring home creatures in a way I did not.

When we were young, Mum rented the same beach house every summer for ten years. It was perfect. On an enormous double block set back behind the eucalypts and tea-trees, it was invisible from the road. Only a few minutes' walk from Shenzi, it was the perfect place for our small family to spend a month every summer. When Mum was heading out, she would send us to Shenzi for Buzz and Grama to give us dinner and sleep over. One light summer's evening, she attached a piece of notepaper to each of our T-shirts with a safety pin. 'WASH ME', it read. Grama's laugh tinkled as she took a photo.

The rented beach house was old. *Old* old. A wide verandah under a corrugated iron roof. Original, flaking linoleum floors and high ceilings. It did not have a television or an inside toilet. The kitchen held a stove I wish I could see now. We were recently watching the excellent time-travelling social documentary, *Further Back in Time for Dinner.* As the 1920s episode aired I leaped forward from the couch: 'That's our beach house kitchen!'

No wonder we had barbecues most of the time.

The most magical time of the day at that house was evening. We would play Kick the Can as the sky turned pink, Mum and friends sitting with sundowners on the verandah, while eucalyptus leaves smoked on the barbie. The heat of the day was still in the ground as us kids raced around the house, hiding in the corners of twisted timber and spider webs. The noise of the gumnut-filled can rattling and skidding across the dirt would be followed with whoops and bellows.

The colour of the sky would be matched in the metallic shell of the Christmas beetles: in the hot January sun they would tuck themselves into the trees and hide in the groundcover. Scarabs with a metallic rainbow sheen.

One summer's afternoon my little brother Jim wandered around the block with a beach bucket, collecting the beetles. He was quiet and meditative, with the deep, lazy rhythm long summer holidays deliver. Hot and still as stones, the beetles filled the plastic yellow bucket all the way up to the top – unmoving and shimmering like petrol reflected in a puddle.

Our bedrooms were next to each other, and much later that night, as the temperature dropped, and Jim and I were falling asleep – a small 'thud'. Then another. Then another. A velvety hailstorm against my bedroom wall, coming from Jim's bedroom.

'Muuuuummm!' The wail of a child – four syllables from one – 'MuuuuUUmmm!'

The Christmas beetles had cooled down. The Christmas beetles had woken up. They filled Jim's bedroom, wings whirring and beetle-scent puffed out from their colourful behinds.

I'm not sure if we used wet towels, but we did manage to get every beetle back in the bucket. As the plastic pail swung over Mum's head, the beetles bounced out into the garden, very cross and very noisy.

Bats and beetles. Mum found some too. In 1965 she was twelve and living in West Africa. She had a secret to show her friend Emma, by a beach just south of Accra. The wind blew in from the sea, smelling of salt. Dry palm fronds crunched under their feet. Emma was irritated, Mum tells us:

'There's nothing here. Tell me what the surprise is.' Emma gets cranky when she can't be the boss. I stop, and she does too.

'Now watch me and do what I do.' I slap the smooth trunk of the palm tree as hard as I can. Both hands, again and again. She does it too, and she slaps even louder than I do.

I shout, 'DON'T STOP DON'T STOP!' We are grinning like wild things.

Now a thousand bats drop in a mass from the canopy above – flapping, rustling, squeaking. We slap and we scream, and we laugh. The noise is around us and inside us. We are bonded now by our secret. It will be waiting for us whenever we return … this magic place. I know it's still there on that empty beach in Ghana.

I was wrong. Touch is as core to remembering as everything else. It is dreamy reflections and warm love. It won't fade if you keep reaching out your hand.

If my hand is not here to hold, it's okay. We don't need three squeezes to share love for one another. Love is in the smooth tree trunks, the flaking lino floors, the glistening slip of a pond-fish and the summer-scented leaf litter. Love is in the memory of touch.

I. Love. You. Too.

Letter Twenty

When you meet a thousand fanciful hells and heavens

I had a psychoanalyst in Hampstead called Tiberius Wolf.

There. That should be the beginning and the end of this letter. If that doesn't compel you to seek out a therapist, I don't know what will. What a wonderful name! What a picture it paints! And what a time to see my (first, and only) psychoanalyst – when I was twenty-four and had barely any psych to analyse.

But maybe that was the problem. I thought I was fine, but I was also unhappy enough to schedule a fifteen-minute cry every weekday morning, with a buffer of time to dry my eyes before applying my make-up. This was when I was working at the cigarette factory agency, so my mascara was already the waterproof kind. Even so, when the weeping started to ooze into other parts of the day, I figured I needed help. Tom, with whom I was now living, agreed. So I sought it on the internet, and because the NHS is miraculous, 24-year-old me didn't have to wait for support, and didn't have to pay for it when I received it.

Mr Wolf worked out of rooms in Frognal, a small pocket of Hampstead, and during our appointments I think I lay on an actual couch. As I commenced our weekly sessions, I would walk up the hill from the Tube in the wintry bite of a London evening. There were red-and-white brick Queen Anne houses on either side, their windows glowing like lamps and tinny with the treble of dinner sounds from within. Each time I made that walk, it was a hunched one. I was huddled against the cold, and the knowledge I had left work 'early'. Which was any time before 7 pm. I was nervous about what that meant for my tomorrow, back at the desk. Tiberius and I only had a handful of sessions together before I chickened out and stopped turning up. I told myself I could no longer manage the early finishes. Weeks after I abandoned our sessions, he finally got hold of me on the phone.

I delivered some spurious excuse about not 'needing' to come anymore. He replied with something along the lines of, 'Well maybe that's a sign you should.'

Lesson #131: What you run away from is often what you actually need.

I went to therapy because I wanted to solve a problem I thought I had. But instead that therapist identified a different one that I didn't realise I had. It was an early lesson that treatment of that kind does not run in a linear fashion and solutions can't be fast-forwarded to. He taught me that the one person you generally thought was great, was probably the one who fucked you up in the first place. And this person could even be yourself. He also taught me that self-diagnosed mental health (such as 'I'm sad because I'm working too hard') is generally inaccurate and often unhelpful.

The final thing my first therapist gave me was permission to acknowledge how ill my homesickness was making me.

*

I grew up with a mother in therapy. She came to it later in life but was always open about how helpful she found – and still finds – it. Mum's therapist, now dead, still makes it into conversation often enough that it's clear how deeply he helped her at a time when she needed it. She describes his room and his words:

> *The faintest smell of his aftershave. The soft click, click of the vertical blinds disturbed by the air-conditioning. I wait for him to respond. I'm used to this and can wait a long time. His eyebrows are up and I hold his gaze.*
>
> *'Well stop telling me it's impossible and fucking well do it.' He looks pleased with himself.*

Lesson #132: Very few things that you are trying to do are truly impossible.

Or, if you're a little older:

Lesson #133: Fucking well do it.

It is normal to have hard times, girl of mine. I've had many periods when my anxiety has kicked me around and held me back. I expect you will have similar experiences, for that is what being a human with a brain is about. The moments make for good dinner party stories. They also help you practise self-awareness, which is one of the highest forms of intelligence.

Lesson #134: Self-awareness is a superpower.

Because of my mother and my experience with therapy, we talk about the process openly with others. But I'm a bit bewildered at how stigmatised mental health treatment still is. I hope by the time you're reading this, my darling, that stain has faded. This letter may still make some people feel a bit blinky and flushed.

I don't think it will do that to you, though. Mainly because your father and I have both been in therapy since before you were born, and we are kinder and nicer to ourselves and each other because of it.

For decades I have worked at the intersection of creativity and commercial pressure. This is not always an environment conducive to happy mental health. Which is why I've had many colleagues with a degree of emotional bruising at some stage. Yet for years I helped reinforce the stigma mental illness attracts by being shy about the therapy required to assist with it.

I have had versions of anxiety, depression, and all the nuances on the spectrum between the two. Yet still, it has taken me a decade to be as open about my psych appointments as I would about any other.

One day, when you were still very small and pink and squashy, I was weeping over our breakfast table. I was weeping because Tom was off to work for another day and we would be alone. I wept a lot back then. I'd become fixated with your sleep routine, and decided sleep school was the only way to 'fix' my tiny baby.

Which is where we went, and they did – but it turns out *I* was the one who needed fixing. You were just a baby.

But you knew that.

After Tiberius had gently suggested I might want to return home, I spent a few years back in Australia focusing my mind and attention on things other than therapy – like getting married and trying to have a baby and grow a career. I didn't meet my next therapist until I attended that five-day sleep school. There I had my first session with a psychiatrist who specialised in women and mothers and people who wept a lot. He suggested that ongoing treatment would be a good idea, and because I'd had two full nights of sleep, the clouds parted long enough for me to agree. Therapy in my early days of motherhood helped me go from loving my baby to being in love with my baby. Something that was a true game-changer.

Yes, sleep school was the beginning of falling deeply in love with you – and it had nothing to do with sleep. Instead, I was given the tools to manage the chaos parenthood brings, tools that allowed me to clear my head enough to see how wonderful being a mother could be. Tools that were given to me by a psychiatrist. He helped me find enough balance to appreciate what you, my baby, *could* do (provide miraculous joy) and what you couldn't (adhere to a robotically strict schedule). Because of all this, sleep school was a successful venture and gifted me a valuable lesson I took into all those disasters I didn't realise were on their way:

Lesson #135: When you can't stop weeping, put your hand up.

Most crucially though, without the homesickness and the parenthood and all the other moments that made me wobbly, I don't think I would've jumped on the therapy train as early as I did. And I'm so pleased that I have sought help early, often and in the face of failure. Because feeling terribly unhappy is not a rite of passage or a lifestyle stage that you should feel concreted to for months (or – my love – years) on end.

Lesson #136: You deserve to be happy.

While you grew through toddlerhood, there were some stop-start years where I only called upon the psychiatrist when things felt particularly weepy. Luckily though, by 2017 I had settled into a routine of monthly appointments, and I started to experience the power of a regular relationship with a therapist. This is when I learned that having a mental health expert 'on tap' is the actual best.

I was diagnosed with cancer on the Wednesday and my monthly appointment was on the Thursday. I went, and took your father along too. Mostly because I kept crying and forgetting what people had said to me.

If I hadn't had a pre-existing relationship with a therapist, I would never have sought help at that crisis point. But boy, I'm glad I had. From that point I saw him weekly, and I credit him for keeping me mostly sane during diagnosis, treatment and the winded shock of PTSD.

Lesson #137: Don't wait for a crisis to call for help.

In the time that I write these letters, many things are accelerating like I've never seen. Some terribly, desperately so – our planet is dying – and some wonderfully, too. Mental health is ever closer to the forefront of people's minds and lives. The stigmas of having a diagnosis attached to mental illness, to be in treatment or taking medication are all being pulled away. And finally, my love – there is an ever-growing acknowledgement of 'triggers' – things that spark your anxiety, or sadness, or any other feeling that is preventing you from thriving.

> *One of the things you learn in that kind of combat is to land in a shell-hole. Quickly.*
>
> *I'll never forget the first time I was under fire; I was accompanying a French colonel, as a sort of aide to him. We were going up to the Front. He was behind me and I was walking ahead, to see that everything was safe, you see. Heavy shelling started, and there was only one shell-hole in the area. It was closer to me, ahead of me on my left. I started for it, and leaped in the air to land in it, but I landed on the colonel. He had a flatter trajectory; he was able to get under me and land first.*
>
> *Here was this elderly gentleman, who had made a study of how to get into a shell-hole quickly. So I myself decided that was something to study and to learn. That's one reason I'm here today.*

During spikes of shock or trauma I've sought air cover under the bombardment of misery. And having therapy and taking medication are valid, reasonable types of 'air cover'. But the most crucial and supportive experience of therapy has been during the 'normal' times.

It's the quiet, persistent work you do on opening up your mind and kneading your psyche that allows the healing and growing to happen. This work allows you to understand how important your triggers are, because they let you to dig a series of shell-holes to dive into when needed. You might not know what they look like at first, but once you've dived into one, you'll make a better study of it for next time.

If you haven't, try it – you might be surprised at what you find.

My shell-holes include:

Moving my body, preferably to the point of sweatiness.

Sitting still and quiet in a place with no other people. It's taken me forty years to establish that loud noises and occasionally other humans (including you, apologies my darling) make me twitchy and anxious. I like the left corner of the terrible sofa we have in the office, looking out the window onto our wonky camellia tree.

Attending therapy on a regular basis, even on the days I don't feel I need it. Particularly on the days I feel I don't need it.

Having Car Picnics. Mum started these when I was at kindergarten. Lilian Cannam Kindergarten was (and still is!) in South Melbourne, but this was long ago when that suburb held dingy milk bars instead of shiny townhouses. We would buy a roast chook and some 'pink drink' and Mum would drive down to the Port Melbourne pier, where we'd watch the boats. *Our* Car Picnics were a tad more bouji (sushi from Brighton, fizzy water for you), but they were still spent looking out over the muted waves of Port Phillip Bay, with conversations ranging far in ways only four-year-olds can extend. Something these two Car Picnics had in common were the mothers (Kate, Ella) would have the children (Ella, you) stick their hands in the air after eating, to be cleaned with wet-wipes.

Cleaning surfaces. Mum has drawn a cartoon about this, in which an elderly woman lies on her deathbed. Her skin puckers around her toothless mouth, open to the concerned-looking family standing in vigil around her. A daughter leans in, listening to her mother's final words. 'She says,' the daughter relays to her siblings, 'she wishes she'd cleaned more surfaces.' This is one of your Gaga's most popular cartoons. I assume most like it because it reinforces the belief that life is too short for Windex and a sponge. But Mum and I know the truth: clean surfaces create a calm, and at least your Gaga and I will never regret grimy Laminex in our final resting places.

Making jokes about bad, sad or mad things. This irritates those around me deeply, but I find it very soothing.

Foot massages with someone I am paying, so I don't feel obligated to chat to them, or return the favour.

Driving while you are 'the Boss of the Music'. You have excellent taste in music and your DJ-ing skills are exemplary for a nine-year-old. You'll wind your way between the Lorax soundtrack through Dua Lipa, back up to Abbey Road and finishing on Whitney before we even cross the Westgate Bridge. We sing loud and long and it gives me fizzes of happiness down my spine.

See? Your psychological shell-holes don't have to be big or impressive or even highbrow. They just have to be there, and close enough for you to dive into when you need them. Also, I hope Jim doesn't mind me knitting a link between near-death in France and a Thai foot massage in my local shopping strip. Something makes me think he'd get a laugh out of it.

A man's mind is a queer stage, dear girl. Its players enter and exit – and their comings and goings and the lines they speak, are in no way controlled by the individual for whom they perform.

> *As a matter of fact, they are extremely likely to be colored – or off colored – by the past experiences of the individual concerned ... I know that at times the eternal theoretical maiden has tripped the boards for me in guises any but saintly – and behind the scenes of my mind, I have lived a thousand fanciful hells and heavens.*

I have been medicated for anxiety, I have been in regular therapy and I have been without either. All approaches have their merits. But I credit a lot of the good work my brain does to the mental pit stops I make at my therapist.

Lesson #138: Find your shell-hole.

Letter Twenty-one

A little party never killed nobody

This family has always loved a party. Generations before me have strung up lights and played music and invented themes and run games and refilled glasses. This is excellent news, because parties are wonderful.

Don't let anyone tell you otherwise. There will come a time when you are expected to eschew parties for more (so-called) sophisticated pursuits, like sitting on sofas in dark corners listening to people talk about work. Defy this tedium! As Buzz said:

> *Virginia and I have always believed that when you have a party you should do something original, something out of the ordinary.*

Reading over Buzz and Virginia's various stories, it's clear that 'out of the ordinary' was a brief they took to heart, all over the world. For many of their parties they organised treasure hunts, with handwritten clues leading to the prize. I've taken this tip on, and can confirm that with sugared-up six-year-olds (much the same as liquored-up thirty-year-olds) it's a guaranteed way to entertain a group of excitable guests. While I've hidden clues in relatively sedate locations like freezer icetrays and sock-drawers, Virginia had her 'frenzied party guests' chasing the family dog for a clue hidden beneath its collar, and crowding into the bathroom to locate the next hint, rolled up and inserted into the toothpaste tube:

One Halloween party, after a hundred rhymed clues had been hidden, the heavens opened and a cloudburst shortly before the arrival of the thirty-eight guests necessitated re-writing and re-hiding clues.

At six-thirty, when I was wandering around half costumed with a glazed look, Jim asked, 'What the hell are you doing?'

'Composing poetry,' says I, 'and can't seem to get the metre quite right.'

Personal barbecuing and rainstorm-soaked clues are eclipsed when Virginia tells us about another treasure hunt at a party in Sierra Leone:

The invitation said we were to wear Hawaiian dress so I spent the day stringing plumeria and bougainvillea blossoms on leis and devising sarongs for us to wear … After a few drinks at the home of the hosts we were all sent out with a list of intriguing objects to bring back.

A live chicken, a bottle of palm wine, some false teeth, a minister's signature.

Jim and I weren't allowed in the same car and ill-assorted foursomes sped off into the tropical night. Also roaring around the roads of Freetown were military vehicles, camouflaged troop carriers and staff cars. They ignored us, we ignored them and only in the morning heard that there had been an attempted coup in this country of unrest.

Lesson #139: If a party is flagging, look for treasure.

The parties that Buzz and Virginia describe seem almost alien in their merriment, with a laissez-faire approach that makes me wonder if all the children were squirrelled away in boxes, or locked in the cars outside. But the opposite was mostly true. The children were there – I just don't think the adults were as bothered by them as much as we are nowadays:

> *We'd dance dreamily to 'Love for Sale' or 'Strangers in the Night', my arms around Jim's neck until I'd feel a pull on my skirt ... it was dawn and the children were up for the day.*

As a child, Virginia was well aware of her own parents' parties, and maybe this is where she received her love of hosting. Jim and Kay were famed for the marvellous gatherings in their Palo Alto home. In particular, their New Year's Eve celebration was so popular that it became a tradition to which their guests held them accountable each year:

> *Each year had a theme carried out in decorations and, often, costumes as well. It was always a noisy party, keeping me awake with the music thumping from the little record player, raucous laughter and one year the sound of a window breaking. Mother crossed the guest responsible for that drunken incident off the list. At midnight Daddy went out in the vacant lot, fired his army pistol into the ground then hurried back inside to play 'Auld Lang Syne' on the piano.*
>
> *Over the fireplace hung huge numerals Daddy had made designating the outgoing year. At midnight the final digit would be replaced, 1933 would become 1934. Mother's good supper was followed by more dancing, more drinking, a few bouts of singing round the piano then:*
>
> *'Happy New Year. Goodnight Male. Goodnight Gladys.'*

'It was the best party ever.'

'Goodnight Birge, goodnight Lucille. Happy New Year!'

I can't tell you about magical parties I've thrown myself. Because I haven't thrown any magical parties myself. This is a regret and one I wished I'd rectified earlier. From the 1990s I have scrapbooks and from the noughties I have Pinterest boards, and even though there are almost twenty years between the two collections – the content is pretty much the same. Fairy lights, deep-green gardens, ivy growing over tables, lanterns bobbing in the gloom. One year, before the internet existed, I even painstakingly transcribed enormous chunks of *The Great Gatsby* into one of the scrapbooks – a recipe for what I envisioned as ~~my twenty-first, my thirtieth,~~ my fortieth party. Look at me, fangirling so hard that I've even dragged a line from the book into this very letter's title. Years later, when Kate Moss threw a 'Beautiful and the Damned' party, I was crestfallen. My party fantasy was Supermodel and Instagram-chic before Instagram existed – and now everyone was doing it better, and before, me. After that, my vision board jumped the shark. And I have no-one to blame but myself (and maybe, my bank account).

Lesson #140: Don't let your dreams stay scrapbooks.

Where I *have* thrown parties, and *good* parties, is when you have been involved. This family doesn't just party as grown-ups, firing pistols and grasping live chickens. We host excellent children's parties.

When Kate turned six, Virginia threw her a Magical Mystery party, and the photographs show a life-sized caravan wagon drawn crudely (sorry, Grama) on brown paper and stuck to the wall.

'Is Angel Food made by real angels?'

'Of course it is. Would you like another piece?'

'COME EVERYONE … sit down and Madame Mystery will tell your fortune!' Mum is talking in her outside voice. The softest frosting, the fluffiest cake. Pin the daisy on the caravan. Jenny is being sick in her own lap and it's pink. Penny still has her blindfold on and is sitting down. Christine is eating more cake, and Mum holds the camera.

'AH yes, WHAT HAVE WE HERE?' Madame Mystery is a real fortune teller, you can tell. She smells like mothballs, has big rings in her ears and many gold bangles. We sit and wait. Ruth is sniffling and wipes her nose on her sleeve. She says in a small sad voice, 'I want to go home.'

'NONSENSE!' shouts Madame Mystery. 'IF YOU GO HOME YOU WON'T KNOW WHAT YOUR FUTURE HAS IN STORE.'

In 1987 Mum threw me *my* own Magical Mystery party. I was also turning six, and while I didn't have a pink Angel Food cake, Madame Mystery made an appearance. This time, she was my aunt, my mother's younger sister. If I recognised her, I didn't let on – to others, or to myself. Madame Mystery looked too exciting to not believe in, and my friends were equally delighted and wary. She arrived towards the end of the party, awash with clanking bangles, headscarves, golden hooped earrings and a pronounced beauty mark under her heavily kohled eyes. We were all bewitched.

Mum also threw me a memorable horror-themed party, which was the first time I remember getting deeply involved in the decorations. We hit up the local video store (look it up) and they gifted us a treasure trove of styrofoam props that they used in their Halloween window displays. We carted bloody limbs and scraggy headstones home and lined the hallway with them. We placed floating plastic eyeballs in the loo and curled a rubber snake deep in the jug of green Cottee's cordial. But the piece de resistance was the seance. Mum and I had carefully recorded a one-sided conversation of a high-pitched woman's voice on cassette (look it up) and slid it into my QFX Shoebox Tape Recorder (look it up). We stuck it under the dining table which was draped in a heavy, floor-length brocade tablecloth and I practised pressing 'Play' and 'Stop' with my toes, all afternoon.

'And how did you die, Ghost of Maude?' I implored, probably quite melodramatically, while my toes blindly danced around beneath the tablecloth.

Click. Clunk.

'I … choked on a chicken booooone!'

I have no idea what my guests thought of the seance, but I had a bloody great time. In fact, my enduring memory of the entire party is not the guests, the gifts or the conversation – it's the preparation, with Mum and your Uncle Jim stuck in.

Lesson #141: If it's your party, throw it for you.

This is why, when you requested your fifth birthday be a 'Magic Faraway Tree' party, I leaped into the planning like Fanny down the slippery-slip. For weeks beforehand I spent nights cutting out paper leaves in different shades of green, and stringing them on to twine. Channelling my grandmother and her caravan, I cut a tree trunk out of brown cardboard and built the foliage up the wall with bunches of green paper, then extended the branches with the leaves. We had toadstools, little forest animals and woodland-themed everything. I'm pretty certain that none of the five-year-olds noticed, and I think I made more enemies than friends out of the other mums.

Lesson #142: No-one likes a mother who tries too hard at craft.

I had fun though. Which is in direct contradiction with Lesson #141. But I couldn't have enjoyed myself too much, because we didn't hold a party at home again for three years.

Your next birthday party was grim, because I was about to start cancer treatment and all the parents had their Sad Eyes on. The party after that, I had finished treatment and was floating on adrenaline at being alive, and fear it wouldn't last. Do you remember that one? We rented out a semi-decrepit dance hall on Glen Huntly Road that was all cracked lino and 'Closing Down Sale' signs. We had a fantastic DJ and discoed our way through the decades. I was two months past my first clear PET scan and still so raw, with fear and relief, every emotion was positively shooting from my fingertips. I wore a gold skirt and you wore disco ball earrings and together we danced so hard that I was laughing and crying at the same time.

That is one of my happiest memories.

Lesson #143: Dance like you may, or may not be, dying.

All good parties have dancing. Unfortunately for you, both your parents are terrible dancers. Strike that. I don't actually think there's such thing as a bad dancer, rather, someone who cares what they look like dancing. Your father cares a lot, I care a little. Cocktails help. Even so, I read Grama's accounts of her parents' dancing and it makes me want to float across parquet flooring with the swish of a gown playing at my ankles.

> *Mother and Daddy loved to dance and they were so good they were often asked to perform exhibition dancing. They gave lots of dancing parties at 640 Middlefield, but often they'd just roll back a corner of the living room rug, put on a record and dance – just the two of them, to 'When I Grow Too Old To Dream'. And sometimes Daddy would ask me to dance, teach me the latest steps. Who wouldn't worship a father who tangoed so superbly: step, step, stepstepstep, hips swivelling before a dip? And who wouldn't envy a mother going off to San Francisco in a neat dark suit and tiny cocktail hat to meet Daddy at the St Francis Hotel for the tea dance?*

Jim taught his daughter to dance, just as he taught his granddaughter to. I told you about Mum dancing with her Grampa when she was sixteen, learning that loose-joined foxtrot, with her feet barely touching the floor:

'Oh Jim.' Grama is delighted as usual. 'How wonderful.'
She looks radiant, stretched out on the chaise lounge, beneath Albert the Alligator, twisting her beads …
'That'll do,' announces Grampa. 'If I'm not mistaken, it's cocktail hour. Who wants to learn how to mix a mountain drink?'

An email exchange, August, 2021:

Ella: Hi Grama, Do you know what JAQ meant when he referred to a 'mountain drink?'
Grama: A mountain drink is lots of bourbon with a bit of water. No ice, you're in the mountains.

Jesus Christ, Jim!

Jim's mountain drink
Bourbon
Water
(No ice, you're in the mountains.)

There's something very evocative about an older man handing me a drink at the end of the day. It feels so old-fashioned, a moment repeated like a black-and-white sitcom. The ceremony of the glass, the ice, the beads of condensation wetting your palm. When we visit Mum and Ross at their house in Point Lonsdale, the ritual of a gin and tonic at the kitchen table has carried on from years earlier, and a block away.

I lift a glass to my dad every time I pour a gin and tonic at Point Lonsdale. He loved to welcome us to Shenzi for the weekend with an icy, refreshing G&T as soon as we walked in the door. I can see the happy, expectant look on his dear face, smell the barbecue, hear his favourite music playing, and remember how it felt to have all the cares of the working week slip away.

I'm told you can still order a 'Mallet' martini in the club Dad joined [when we first lived in Melbourne], and it will be served to my dad's exact 1959 instructions. In those days the American-style, knock-out strength martini hadn't reached Australia. Dad soon fixed that. He developed a reputation amongst his most seasoned Aussie mates for mixing a killer martini.

They named it the Mallet for good reason.

The Mallet martini

Fill a medium glass with ice chunks (Buzz preferred to freeze an un-sectioned tray of solid ice, and break it up with a pick).

Pour two ounces of good gin over the ice, then a bare whisper of dry vermouth.

Stir, and drop in two stuffed green olives on a toothpick.

Drink, and wait for your gums to go numb.

Lesson #144: Be careful of any cocktail mixed by an American.

Cocktails are not just for numbing the gums of seasoned Australians. They help at dinner parties too – getting guests in the mood, and then sustaining them when the food doesn't. Your father and I hosted some friends at our first home in Australia, a rental in Prahran with floating stairs and frosted glass tiles. After the Belsize flat, it felt enormous and clinical, like we were playing grown-ups. And, it turns out, we were. We did not know how to roast a chicken, cook vegetables to accompany it or do anything other than continually open bottles and serve bowls of crisps to our increasingly hungry (and increasingly drunk) guests.

We were, I'm pleased to see, in good company. In Buzz and Virginia's first home, also a rental, the newlyweds decided to host their first dinner. There was only one problem:

> *I couldn't cook.*
>
> *Our first guests were my parents whom I trusted to put up with my weakness. Jim mixed martinis just the way Daddy liked them and we sat under our willow tree on our lawn, playing host and hostess.*
>
> *'What are we having for dinner?' asked Mother.*
>
> *'Leg of lamb,' I proudly answered.*
>
> *'How's it going?'*
>
> *'Oh, I haven't put it in yet. The recipe said half an hour.'*
>
> *'I think it might mean half an hour per pound, dear.'*
>
> *Lots of martinis were consumed, almost enough to make the raw lamb edible.*

Grama's dinner parties improved and I remember sitting at her table in Shenzi, the lamb cooked perfectly and only one Mallet per adult. That was better.

Enduring memories of our parent's dinner parties at number 38 are of the mornings after the nights before. My brother and I would creep down with all the excitement of children awake too early on Christmas morning. The dining table would be set like a Caravaggio, almost otherworldly in the blue morning light. We would survey the scene like a tiny pyjama-ed forensic team: small wine glasses with red stains at the bottom, overflowing glass ashtrays tainting the house with the smell of what I now associate as the Olden Days, strawberry stems and cheese cracker crumbs, crumpled paper clues to some mysterious parlour game that would have been produced after midnight. And, the treasure we were looking for: hidden like Easter eggs among the tableware and linen – a glimmer of muted gold.

The Ferrero Rocher.

It would be a thrill to sift through the detritus to find a chocolate. Like Charlie Bucket, most of the golden glimmers were disappointingly empty wrappers – but one in three … jackpot! Sated, full of hazelnut and chocolate, we'd retire to the couch and cartoons until our parents emerged for the clean-up.

Lesson #145: Do the dishes before you go to bed.

Mum continued to throw dinner parties after she became single again, but the epic ones, the 1980s ones, really produced the goods: chocolate, parents sleeping in, and – in my father's case – fractured chairs. A tall man, my dad left a wake of splintered wood across Melbourne for over a decade. He had a habit of swinging back on chairs, as the night wore on. His 2.6-metre frame was not suited to such activities:

> *Woodsmoke, aftershave, voices bray over the music. I hear it before anyone else does because I know the sound well. It's the sound a century-old dining chair makes just before it implodes. A dry, rending wheeze … and I'm already reaching out to stop it. But I'm too late.*
>
> *The chair legs splay, his legs fly up and a gout of wine arcs over his head into the fireplace. He takes too long getting to his feet, not saying much, looking surprised. We are all quiet now and the music plays on.*
>
> *Now everyone is whooping and laughing, even the woman who lives in the house, who has prepared this dinner and paid for this chair.*

One thing the pandemic has taken from us is the opportunity to throw a party. As we near two years in and out of lockdown, the tally marks on the walls of our homes have stretched far beyond what we expected. I don't want to even guess how much longer we will be in this Hokey-Pokey of isolation. One of the things this has taught us, however, is how to snatch a party from thin air. Catering, musicians costumes, are gone – for now. Instead, we gather when and how we can.

With Kay in Washington and Jim serving out his time in France, it seemed he was also managing to find some party in between the frontline and the retreating enemy:

> *I happened to ride over to [—] where Capt. Pat is stationed and told him that you remembered him in your letter. He seemed genuinely pleased. He's a lucky dog – has the best billet in the district – an old chateau with a piano and silver cutlery and – what is almost unbelievable – a real toilet in the house.*
>
> *I stayed for dinner and they had two kinds of champaigne [sic]. Oofff! I wish I had a phonograph record of the conversation. Nobody understood anybody else but there was an abundance of champaigne and international goodwill, both of which flowed freely.*

Lesson #146: Take your party where you can find it.

Earlier this year Dad and his wife hosted us at his home outside Melbourne. It had been a stinking hot day, contrary to the freezing one we had last seen Daylesford in, six months and two lockdowns prior. The novelty of sharing a meal around a table was still there. Their courtyard was glowing in the candlelight, a balmy night steaming quietly as the sun set before us. Their cottage garden bristled with herbs and vegetables. Prawns were barbecued over a drum-fire. There was an abundance of goodwill and excellent food, Dad did not break any chairs. It was a lovely little party.

Letter Twenty-two

Explosions

Sometimes, life blows up.

You will not expect it; you will not know it's coming. It will destroy and maim and terrorise but – sadly, unimaginably – life will go on. This is a letter that will tell you about times when our lives have been blown up. Shaken down, exploded on and broken apart. If we were a different type of family, a group of people who chose to see the world through a different lens, this might be the letter about Bad Luck.

Shall we try that coat on for size? Here is my own stab, at a letter about our Bad Luck Family:

Jim's family moved to California and built a home, just in time for the largest earthquake in living memory to shake them from their foundations.

Later (but not too much later) when Jim was fighting in the war, he found himself at the intersection of German machine guns and artillery. Jim nearly died from shrapnel wounds in the ensuing attack.

A wounded war veteran, Jim had three children with his wife, Kay. It was their daughter, Virginia, who contracted polio. At the time, Virginia was a young bride and mother, and her husband, Buzz, wept at the table when he considered his children's motherless future. Only recently Buzz himself had avoided death by the narrowest of clerical errors, surviving another war when the other five officers he started out with did not.

Virginia survived, and with Buzz also had three children. Her daughter Kate was a single mother for longer than she was anything else. Kate had two children, one of whom, her daughter, was diagnosed with a rare and advanced cancer when she was a young mother.

Bad luck, tragedy, misfortune followed this family through generations.

It doesn't work, does it? Because that is not our family. It may be our story, in some collection of words, but you and I both know that that story is not us.

Lesson #147: You are not the sum of your stories.

No, we are – do you remember? – we are a group with a tendency to attract luck, trauma, glitz and knocks. Things explode. We explode back.

I was eleven years old when the earthquake came, in 1906.

Bang. 5.40 in the morning. April 18, 1906. Fortunately, everybody was not out on the streets.

About 8.00 in the morning I said to my parents, 'I think I'll go uptown and see what kind of damage has been done.' Now my father said, 'No, son, just a minute'... But my mother said, 'Let the boy go uptown. It's the only way we can find out what's going on!'

Jim's family had relocated from Maryland to California in time for them to witness what was the worst earthquake in the state's history. His father had recently finished building their new house, and the tremors took it off its foundations, as if shaken by an enormous explosion. Jim was eleven and he saw things he would never forget:

> *When I got about three blocks to where [the residential section] was built up, I couldn't go in the street, because [it] was full of destroyed facades … the street was full of bricks. And the houses looked like doll houses, all rooms vacant. You could look into them. Here were beds with one foot out, [just] hanging out of the aperture.*

I was twenty-four years old when the bombs came, in 2005.

Bang. 9.47 in the morning. July 7, 2005, when the bus exploded at the end of my road. The bomb opened the double-decker up like an unfolded lily, its red petals reaching out in a way you should never see.

I didn't know that the noise was a bus blowing up. I didn't know the deep 'boom!' was the sound of people dying. Of course I didn't. At the time, when you are in the midst of the very time, you never do.

Lesson #148: You won't know you're in the explosion until afterwards.

It was early Thursday morning and I had arrived at work. When I was writing this to you I discovered an email I sent to my family in Australia on the same day, much much later – once we'd all found our way home. If you'd asked me about this morning before I'd found the email, I'd have told you I'd probably been in the office kitchen making a cuppa, maybe I had checked emails first. I didn't remember the detail of that morning, until I read about it.

I wasn't making a cuppa – I was calling my boyfriend and my mother and wondering what the news really meant when they said, 'power surges'. I'd also forgotten that the bus that was blown up had been diverted, and so had exploded at my bus stop.

Lesson #149: Your memory can have a knack of losing itself, to protect you.

The first shift in energy from the day being Normal to something Not Being Quite Right was the news reports of those 'power surges' in the Tube. When you're living in an Event you realise how messy and uninformed live news is. It isn't until the analysis and hindsight kicks in that a timeline can be created. It made my skin feel itchy, to be watching the news and seeing the anchors look bewildered. There was no autocue.

Once the bomb went off, the phones went down and I couldn't get through to Tom. He had been on the Tube when the explosions started, but just happened to remain ahead of them. Tom rode the carriages ahead of the explosions like Buzz swimming far out while the tidal wave swelled beneath him.

Having no phones: that was the second shift. When I couldn't get a hold of Tom, I fretted. I didn't know he was safe. We didn't know if there had been more bombs, and I didn't want to consider what that all meant. I briefly contemplated running through London to find him, but those energy shifts were happening all around and moving beneath us. What was safe and expected thirty minutes ago was suddenly not safe at all. Then different language was starting to filter through the news. Bombs. Terrorists. Attacks. Six years after 9/11 this seemed at once shocking yet expected.

And then the bus blew up near the office and I wouldn't have been able to get to Tom if I tried. Police arrived, sealing us into the building with yellow emergency tape. We all herded down to the basement kitchen and someone dragged the metal gates across the windows. We didn't know what to do; we didn't know what was happening. History hadn't tidied up the story for us yet –

were there planes? Were there people in the streets who wanted to hurt us? Would everything change? Questions were asked that now seem silly, but then seemed completely reasonable.

> *The Sunday in 1941 when the Japanese bombed Pearl Harbor, Siddy and I sat in the back seat of the Cadillac with [our dog] Jack. We'd been on a picnic and as Daddy drove, Mother turned on the radio to listen to the Charlie McCarthy show. We heard the stark news in disbelief. Mother thought of the boys, they'd be in this war, Daddy combined this knowledge with his memories of the mud, blood and gas of his war.*
>
> *Siddy and I looked at each other wide-eyed, scared. Would the Japanese bomb us? Would everything change?*

We sat and waited and watched the bloody, sooty, stunned people emerge from Underground via the TV. I got hold of Tom: he was okay.

I told him, 'I'm okay.'

I spent most of the day in the basement messaging relatives in Australia to say: 'I'm okay. I'm okay.'

We were eventually allowed to leave, and we walked past the bus. The big red bloom – it is wretched to see metal twisted and ugly. Wretched to know that it held death, so recent it still felt warm. I kept the bus in the corner of my eye as we skirted the perimeter. I tried not to see the white sheets over small things. Surely too small to be bodies. But we knew what they were.

To the pub. Always the pub. In Britain, you go to the pub. This time, the blue pub with the timbered tables down the cobbled lane. It was a mild evening and the crowds were heaving. Beer, beer, shouting, *laughing*, hysteria. Writing these words, I know you'll think it sounds uncouth. But it wasn't. Reading the letters from Jim to Kay, as he fought his way through France and into Belgium, there are jokes. Some of them make me wince, but I won't shake my head. Trauma and shock come out in laughter, black and bleak – but laughter nonetheless.

> *There is much to laugh at in this war. A man I saw who got excited in a gas shell attack and put his rubber dispatch case over his head, thinking it was his mask.*
>
> *He was laughable, but very dead.*

I cried when I saw Tom, and then we all drank to ignore the TV screens in the corner showing bandaged faces. When it was clear we couldn't stay out any longer, we joined all of the people moving reverentially through the darkened streets of London. Many women had their shoes in their hands, heels not suitable for nearly five kilometres of trekking. There were no buses, there was no Tube, there didn't seem to be any cars at all. Just thousands of feet, slowly padding their way home.

When you've been exploded-on, it's hard to see straight ever again. The morning after we walked home with the rest of London, Tom and I steeled ourselves to step back onto a London bus. The Tube was still closed, but the buses were running and we needed to get to work. My stomach was in knots when we boarded, I was too clammy to enjoy the lack of crowds and the availability of prime top-deck seats. We gripped hands as we sat on the garish upholstery and as Tom busied himself with his BlackBerry, I searched the faces of those around me for a sign that I should be scared. And there it was – a black backpack sat unwatched under a seat across the aisle. I didn't stop to think.

'Excuse me!?' I was calling out, my voice was high.

'Excuse me … whose bag is this?' Almost shouting.

A harried young woman lurched back and clutched the bag – it had slipped from under her seat to the one behind. Everyone looked at me, at her, at the bag. I was so cross.

'Be careful!' I said, quieter this time. Eyes wide under beetled brows, staring into hers, imploring her to feel the fear I was. '*Be careful.*'

Lesson #150: Nothing looks the same after a trauma. Be prepared to refocus.

> *Miss Powell is my nurse, and she's a peach. If she weren't about forty years old, I'd fall in love with her immediately. Has a lot of brown hair, and brown eyes that laugh all the time. The other night she took me over to Maiden Lane to see the fireworks. The display was fine. Rockets, and set pieces, and gun fire imitation smoke barrages, against one of the parks that occur so unexpectedly here in London.*
>
> *The ladies and civilians clapped and cheered [the fireworks], but as I looked around me at the other chaps in uniform, I found them gazing with fixed eyes at the lights and smoke that flashed and died through the blackness and tracery of tree trunks. They were thinking, as I was, of other nights when rockets soared, and flashes lit the darkness. Don't think I'll ever enjoy fireworks.*

Enjoy the blurry days.

Enjoy not worrying about things like unattended bags or expansively stretching fireworks or an ache in your groin that you weren't sure was there before.

*

I was thirty-six years old when the cancer came, in 2018.

Bang. 1.30 in the afternoon. April 18, 2018. Although it wasn't so much of a bang as a series of sad whimpers that built up and up and up until I found myself howling into Tom's armpit at 11 pm, trying not to wake my five-year-old daughter in the next room. That was you. I hope you didn't hear me. I'm sorry if you did.

The thing about cancer is there's no Hollywood moment where some bloke in a white coat holds your hand and tells you gently, 'You have … The Cancer.' I mean, maybe they do, but not with me and my bottom. Instead, April was a collapsing domino tower of horribly surreal conversations where I ended wondering: 'How should I be sitting while she tells me this?' and: 'I'm going to wait for Tom to leave the room before I start crying, I don't want to upset him.'

2018 was our own personal earthquake, a private explosion that opened up our lives in an ugly way, like the bus. It was mid-autumn and I had found a small lump on my bikini line. In less than a fortnight I went from having a 'likely hernia' to a biopsy-confirmed squamous cell carcinoma, up my bum. I had anal cancer and it was in my lymph nodes. That, as they say, escalated quickly.

I'm so grateful you were not aware enough to understand the horror the initial diagnosis days brought upon myself and your father. I could not protect myself, but I could protect you. Or I could then. You were a term into your first year at school and your first question when we eventually told you that I 'was sick in my bottom', was, 'Do you have worms, Mama?'

I can honestly say: I never lied to you. But we rarely told you the grown-up truths either.

Lesson #151: Sometimes it is okay to protect someone from the whole truth.

It became a badge of honour and requirement for me to ensure we kept you insulated in a swaddle of serenity. I wish I'd had Grama's tips for placing oneself in that same swaddle, when the explosion goes off. In the early 1950s, she too nearly died of an illness she did not expect:

> *We weren't even thirty, madly in love, healthy, happy, with two wonderful children. Everything was perfect. Until I got polio.*

> *At first I diagnosed it as the flu but Jim thought the doctor should come up and look at me. Much to my surprise I was whisked into the Huntington Hospital in Pasadena for tests. I couldn't hold any food and had a splitting headache. They did a spinal tap which was very painful and indicated I [was positive] …*
>
> *Psychologically I was protected by a curious serenity, insulated from terror. I wasn't upset but, of course, Jim was devastated. He visited, we spoke into microphones and blew kisses through a glass panel [and] I kept him informed as to the progress of the paralysis in my legs.*
>
> *He went back up the hill, thinking as he drove of how he could modify the house to accommodate a wheelchair.*
>
> *Our life would certainly be different now, not the dream future we'd taken for granted. My neighbour, returning the children, found him with his head down on the kitchen table, sobbing.*
>
> *The Salk and Sabin vaccines weren't available yet though there was some thought that gamma globulin might help. Jim had this given to both the children but not himself – it was too expensive.*

I can't imagine Buzz's fear: his wife, the mother to his children, filtering her love through tinny microphones and glass panels. The fear that not only she would go, but maybe one – both – of their children too. That he tried to protect them before himself, like any parent would.

Lesson #152: We would do anything for you. Anything.

The thing about getting sick as a mother is your first and last thought to bookend every day is your child. You. *You* were my thought. In the darkest moments of cancer I had two small voices, circling one another like an interior yin/yang:

'At least it's not her. At least she's well.'

And, *'Oh, please let me be around for her. Please, let me live.'*

Those narratives – Gratitude and Pleading – nibbled at each other's tails for months and years.

April 18 was also the day that we asked Mum and Ross to meet us at home. Straight from the GP appointment, we had picked you up from school. Your father popped you in his car and took you home. I got back in the other car, drove around the corner and parked under a big gum tree. My stomach sat up in my chest and my lungs between my ears. I called Mum, because I couldn't have this conversation in front of you. As she sat in my kitchen, I sat in my car, and I told her what the doctor told me. I started to cry.

It sounded different from any of the cries I'd had before. It was low, guttural and full of fear. The two narratives started up again. This time, a Rational one (*you're fine, it can't be that bad, you need to sort out work, is your health insurance all up to scratch? Gee this is going to seem hysterical when they tell you they've made a silly mistake …*) and the other, the other train of thought that didn't run in full sentences or even words (*ohhh you're a mama, you need to be a mama for this little girl. She's five. Not now. Anything. I'll do anything. What can I promise? Who can I bargain with? No, no, no, no*).

I expect there comes a time in everyone's life when you realise your own mother can't make it all better. That was mine. Mum said all the right things. She promised me everything would be okay. And I couldn't believe her.

It's moments like that that stay with you.

*

I was thirty-seven years old when the pandemic came in 2020.

Bang. March 16, 2020. We were told to go home and stay home and the pessimists among us (hi) thought we might be home for an entire month.

In the beginning, the whole world was locked down, but fear and mass solitude kept us connected. Each night we watched as cases spiralled across the news bulletin maps. We were living through a collective trauma, existing in a time that we already knew would be replayed to others, endlessly, through books, films – and media that doesn't even exist yet.

But like the explosions that came before, history hadn't tidied up the story for us so far. It still hasn't. As I write, we continue to breathe history that doesn't yet have an end. The world hasn't done this for a hundred years. And even then, they didn't do it like this. Not this isolated, but this connected. Not this unprecedented, but this over-informed. And never – never – at this speed. It feels like every month that passes, another First tumbles down and we continue to stand at the front line of history in the making. It is not a nice feeling.

In late August of 2020, we marked the nineteenth week of cumulative lockdown. Our city had been under its first curfew since World War II but I was driving after sunset. A visit to the pharmacy had allowed me my first after-hours foray into the world, for months and months. As I slowed to turn back onto our road, the final gloom melting into the deeper night, I saw a mother and her daughter crossing before me.

Mother, masked, hunched, gripping her child's hand. Girl, wet-washed-hair and pyjamas beneath her dressing gown. How incongruous. Maybe, in the Beforetimes, it would have been a slightly eccentric family duo out for a late-winter walk. But now. This time – oh, my sweet. It hit me in my belly. It was a work-weary mother hurrying her child home after dark, because walking her daughter through the winter wet Melbourne streets was all that was left to do.

The second year of the pandemic has brought a different sensation. We are more isolated than before, as different parts of that world map splinter off and manage their catastrophe in their own way. And in our own country it's the same: race, class, religion, social beliefs – we are all splintering. Splintering behind our screens as we hurry back into our homes.

The rolling lockdowns are, arguably, more tortuous than the first long one. It is a roller-coaster through treacle. We are heavy. We are tired. Every time will be more depleting. Every time will get easier. That's the sad part. That's the hopeful part. We have barely enough time to take our breath after the slow gut-punch of one press conference before another comes. We have less than a month to compress and decompress. We are weary accordions, wheezing through monotony and unknowing and repetition and unease.

My girl, your father and I are using every trick to get you through this lonely, sad time for a young child with no siblings. Fresh air, moving our bones, saltwater, belly breathing, sleeping, crying. Lots of screens. No screens. Nutritious, wholesome food. Sugary food that hugs our tummies. All of it and none of it works.

If we can carry anything from this pandemic it is this: life will never be normal again. And that's okay.

Lesson #153: If you are ever lucky enough to live in a boring time, appreciate it.

Bang. 11.15 in the morning. August 26, 2020.

'Can you wait outside, mate? I need to talk to your mum quickly.'

I had done this enough times to know when a doctor is scared. No-one likes telling a young mother that she is seriously ill. No-one likes telling that young mother that her daughter might be the same. It was a routine check-up on your eyes, your pupils had not been sitting right, and now here we were again. In the car afterwards when you looked at me questioningly I told you, you might be getting glasses.

My Gratitude voice came back to me from 2018: *'At least it's not her. At least she's well.'*

*

It was Tom who took you to the MRI at the Royal Children's: there was no amount of Valium and ice cream to keep me from breaking down as they put you in that tube. That was my cross to bear, that was *my* tube. You did not belong in that donut-ring of fear.

You see, I was as brave as a soldier when I was running the gamut of the 'you might bes'. That's the first type of terror. It's a quiet trauma, one that is slowly boiling your bones. A muted one. A private pain: 'You might be. You might have.' I knew that terror, I could hold it.

But the next one, was a screaming missile of gruesome fear. She might be. *Your daughter* might be. Your daughter might have. It was a spiked one. I thought I knew terror. I was the smug cancer chick who made sweary jokes about feeling mortal. But this time, it was my only child. My daughter. You.

She might have this syndrome. It's likely. This syndrome might mean she has.

I have had cancer.

I have had loved ones die.

I have lived through bombs and betrayal and brutality, but that. *That.*

Nothing has ever filled me with more terror than that.

Lesson #154: There is always a bigger mountain lion.

You didn't. Your brain MRI was clear and there was no tumour, which meant no syndrome, which meant your pupils are just … that way.

And you still don't need glasses.

*

I don't tell you these stories of fear and horror to terrorise you, my sweet. I tell them to you because we survived. All of us did.

Terrible things happened to us and we lived, we skirted, shifted, closed on ourselves and then opened up again. And then we died. But even so – do you remember your Gaga's lesson?

Lesson #155: Things will get better again.

As much as it hurt to not believe my mother at the time, when she told me that 'everything will be okay', I can now tell you the same thing. I am dead, you might die, there may be hideous, horrible, gruesome terror around the next twenty corners. But I can promise you that as long as you have breath, you have hope that something, somewhere, will be better again soon.

Letter Twenty-three

Never give up on magic

Once upon a time Pinky and Greenie were flying along, flying along, flying along and what do you s'pose they saw? They saw a little girl with black hair and dark eyes, sturdy legs sticking out from beneath her pinafore. They saw a blonde-haired child with blue eyes as big as a doll's, wearing her brother's hand-me-down corduroy trousers. They saw a dark-haired girl with freckles on her nose, and two warts on her left hand.

Dear Ella,
We're sorry you have a cold! We both had one last month, but are better now. We come and watch you every night, and make sure you have sweet dreams! We love you so much, even your warts. Don't worry about them, they will go away. You are a beautiful girl, you know! Our house looks a bit like this. It's in a BIG apple tree not far away. It's very cosy inside and safe from cats (we don't like cats). Thanks for the surprises, we'll take them home. We'll kiss you goodnight and go now,
Love from
Pinky and Greenie xxoo

I wrote many letters when I was younger. Mostly to two fairies, called Pinky and Greenie. I knew about them because they had visited my mother when she was little, and visited her mother when *she* was little:

> *… my pre-school years [would find me] confiding in my imaginary friend 'Jersey' or listening to Mother's stories of 'Once upon a time Pinky and Greenie were flying along, flying along, flying along and what do you s'pose they saw?'*

Pinky and Greenie have continued to visit our family – which you know, because they have been flying into your room for years now. You write letters to them, and they reply. Why have they chosen to follow our family around the world, for nearly one hundred years? It could be, because this family has always lived with a puff of magic dust in the periphery. But this isn't luck, or coincidence, oh no.

Lesson #156: You make your own magic.

As a family, we have conjured our own magic for decades. We have Pinky and Greenie. Father Christmas, of course. There are gypsies and ghosts. And castles and elves and dragons and kings. All these magical characters have had one thing in common: they have helped us through the hardest of times. The mind is the most powerful thing we all have at our disposal, and it can protect you and keep you in such a special way. Our family magic has allowed us to witness pain through a glittered filter.

When Jim was fighting in Europe, he knew how important this framing could be:

> *Do you know, Lady, this whole thing – all of it – strikes me as the living out process of some grown up fairy tale. Remember when you were a little tyke how you used to dream of working out*

some fantasy with yourself – always yourself – as the Beeyootiful Princess? And now, with me, the romances I have read and the dreams I have dreamed are nothing more than fairy tales revised to suit my apparent age. I'm a boy still, Kay girl, and I like to laugh at things and pat myself on the back for laughing and glory in it.

Lesson #157: Laugh at the glory of dreams and fairytales.

I wasn't aware of 'the Game' until you and Gaga had been playing it for some months. In the front room of number 38, you had both created intricate worlds. It's my mother who taught me the power of imagination, and how magic follows anyone who uses that power. She's always been wonderful at that: painting a picture in the mind of the most unusual and wonderful scenarios. In your preschool years, you and your grandmother spent days together in a universe of your own making. A world of evil witches throwing curses, brave maidens vanquishing dragons, and dashing princes throwing fabulous parties. You both spent many afternoons in those two front rooms, mixing new memories and painting them all over the walls of the house I grew up in. Mum allowed me a glimpse at this, recently:

'COME MY DRAGONS. I SUMMON YOU BY ALL THE FORCES OF MY MIGHTY KINGDOM.'
I stand transfixed. WHUMP – WHUMP – WHUMP.

They drop in great lazy swoops from the battlements. Sunlight flashes off their scales in glints of copper and green.

'Your Highness, we must leave immediately. I have word that their armies gather beyond the Dark Forest.'

She is fierce and formidable, afraid of nothing – winged or not. I bow before her.

Lesson #158: The magic of fierce women is that they create fierce women.

Those two front rooms were the same ones that Father Christmas visited me in, each childhood December. The extraordinary excitement of waking on Christmas morning and knowing that He had been inside my actual house was so visceral, I still remember the stomach-drop of excitement a split-second after my eyes opened. The thrill of coming down the stairs, rounding the corner and seeing gifts beneath a tree where last night there had been nothing, is the very centre of that kind of magic. Luckily for my brother and me, Mum was less strict about the Christmas morning procession than Jim and Kay were with Virginia and her brothers:

> *Christmas morning was ruled strictly, by tradition. No-one was allowed to peek through the glass doors into the living room and we must follow normal morning routine. Shivering with cold and excitement I fumbled my way into my clothes and appeared at the breakfast table in such a state of agitation I couldn't possibly swallow a bite. Daddy finally relented, left the dining table to light the fire and turn on the Christmas tree lights. As we assembled, in order of age, to march into the living room I could see the glow from the tree and the flickering firelight silhouetting the stockings we'd hung there the night before, now exquisitely lumpy.*

Lesson #159: Yes, Father Christmas is real.

I've told you I worked with Father Christmas, but have I told you how doused in magic the job was? Of course, there was the anxiety in the eyes of some visitors that I told you about earlier. But the overwhelming, candy cane-dusted majority were cause for genuine Christmas cheer.

In my time at Myer's Santa Land I witnessed many Christmas miracles. I saw surly seventeen-year-old boys transform, eyes lighting up like their mother's flashing earrings as I reintroduced them to Father Christmas. I saw young children ask for heartbreaking things, like 'bring Daddy home from hospital' – but I also saw them thank the big man for 'making our family really happy'. It was a sugar plum-fuelled roller-coaster and I loved it.

My job as Santa's Helper taught me to weave magic into the everyday, and that empathy still has a role in a commercially minded world. I think that job set me up better for my eventual career in advertising than any work experience or university degree did. Smoke, mirrors, flashing lights and banging doors. Being a Santa's Helper and an Advertising 'suit' was very similar. All of it prepared me – Pinky and Greenie. Gypsies and ghosts. You.

We've all had brushes with holders of magic. Those who can create something from nothing are the most magical of them all. In 1966, Kate was doing what children have done for centuries: mooching around their parents' parties and stealing chips from the snack board. However *this* party was at Walt Disney's house in Palm Springs – and guess who took her for a ride around the grounds?

The leather seat is wet with dew in the sharp, cold desert air. Should I wipe it with my sweater? I freeze.

'Here Princess, let me do that,' says Walt (… Walt Disney! …) and pulls a red handkerchief out of his pocket. He starts the jalopy, hands me the steer-lever and we bounce down the driveway. He sweeps his arm high.

'THIS is what I come here for – the DESERT SKY.'

We loop around for a thumbs-up from the security guard and then turn onto the road. Sand and cactus, boulders and tumbleweed flash by the headlights. The sky is a cobalt-blue sari, sequinned with gold. The stars are fireworks, snap frozen.

We pull up at the front door, I'm lifted from my seat and set lightly down like a dancer. 'Now, let's see these latest drawings of yours,' he says. And we walk back through the door to the grown-up party inside.

I used to wish on every star I saw. I've mentioned that haven't I? The first of each night, when it was twinkling like that snap-frozen firework. Just because, as I told you, the day I was diagnosed with cancer I stopped wishing on stars doesn't mean I don't believe in magic. I believe in every part of the magical, imaginative world you joined when you were born into this family. The thing about magic and fairytales is they can absorb any amount of real life you can throw at them.

Lesson #160: If you look at dirt and can see glitter, life will always be sparklier.

Imagination is another superpower, and you were born with more than your fair share, my darling girl. It's a legacy passed to you from a long line of wonderers and it will do you well, like it did Jim, summoning Kay to the middle of France.

> *You come to me many times these days, my dear, for I'm lonesome and I'm blessed – or cursed – with an active imagination. Not that I see you in any particular place – when I want you in Washington, or in Camp Lewis, I have to build the picture with you in it. But when you come to me, uncalled, you come just as yourself, with no background at all, at all.*

My great-grandmother Kay made her own wishes. I did not know this until I had almost finished this letter to you. But then Kay's words appeared in an email, scanned in by her 96-year-old son, across the world mid-pandemic and that is magic. Because … read this; read what words appeared in my inbox:

> *My father's illness cast a shadow over all of our lives. I remember for years wishing on the first star of evening that my father got well.*

Kay did not get her wish. Her father died in 1918. My wish, however, came true:

> *Starlight, star bright, first star I see tonight, I wish, I wish … to have a healthy baby.*

This was my single wish, over and over, mouthed into the sky. A plea, a promise and a bargain all wrapped into one. I did not pray to a god, but I sure did wish upon a star.

Lesson #161: There's a difference between magic and 'magical thinking'.

You are the most magical thing in my life. Because you are a miracle.

It was my thirtieth birthday, and Tom and I were dining in a special restaurant hidden among the tea-trees and salt marshes of the Bellarine Peninsula. We had even booked a bed and breakfast in the nearby town, trying to make the night 'special', in a time when milestones felt like millstones, shouldered without a child. Queenscliff didn't have Ubers in 2011. A friendly local taxidriver took us there and back. He had a moustache and asked if we had kids.

'No, not for us,' I said. Tom's fingers crept over mine in the back seat, and we held hands as the moonlight flashed through the knotted branches.

After dinner, we arrived back at the nineteenth-century guesthouse, with its red bricks and wraparound first-floor verandah. Tom felt for the key. I felt for the key. The key felt for us, because it was upstairs in our hotel room, and we were outside in the dark. I considered the phone call I'd have to make to my mother, at her home, in her bed, not placed very conveniently for the midnight safety dash we needed.

Thirty years old and tipsy in a country town.

'Mum? We're locked out. Can you come get us?'

It's a quirk of the local architecture in those parts that the upstairs verandahs have external timber staircases. As I was about to hit 'Call' on my phone, Tom noticed that our guesthouse had one of these sets of stairs, and its gate was unlocked. Tom climbed the stairs and yes – our room was the only one with access to the verandah. And yes – we had left the French doors unlocked. And yes – we made it inside, to our key and our room. And yes – that was the night you were conceived.

So your existence was nearly thwarted by a lost key and the temptation of an Italian adventure. Like I said, you are a miracle – in a thousand ways more than one.

The final magic in our family is the one most sought after in tales of glittering broadswords and fairy castles: everlasting life.

There is a proverb often attributed to the ancient Egyptians about the power of speaking the name of the dead. David Eagleman, American neuroscientist and author, captured it as such:

> *There are three deaths. The first is when the body ceases to function. The second is when the body is consigned to the grave. The third is that moment, sometime in the future, when your name is spoken for the last time.*

These letters are filled with the names of the dead. Let's place twenty cents into each mausoleum and keep telling stories as long as we can. It's time for us to begin our goodbyes, to acknowledge who is gone, while we keep them alive by sounding out their names.

Say it with me out loud: 'James. Jim. Daddy. Grampa.'

Lesson #162: There's magic in your words.

Letter Twenty-four

Sounds

'Sound' is not just about rock'n'roll 'n' romance. It is not disco balls and starlight. There are sounds that tug on our heart just as firmly as music does. Before we start singing, let's start by listening:

> *The window of my billet stands open upon the pleasant village street … Frenchmen, who live across the way, mingle their many murmurous voices in comment upon the playing of an orchestra in the adjoining barn. The tune is one which has to do with Irish eyes and is played as a serenade to a French maiden on a Hawaiian instrument by an undersized Italian who is a very good American soldier. Therefore the ensemble merits the success which it seems to be achieving.*

Jim could enjoy the open window, because the guns weren't yet sounding. Two months later he was surrounded by a barrage of warfare.

> *It was here, on the day before our attack, that I had my first look at no-man's-land, and it made an impression on me that I will*

> *never forget. No sign of a human being – merely a great, desolate waste of torn earth, with fragments of trees and wreckage strewn about on its surface. The prevailing impression was stark, dreary and dead – a dead earth, like part of the dead moon.*

There's something about the conjunction of silence and sound that makes me feel uncomfortable.

Virginia told us about the sound of the 'twang of rigging on masts' that accompanied their last American home. That hollow 'twang' of flagpole metal is so specific, and makes me feel oddly anxious when I hear it ... but ask me when I have, and my ears draw a blank with my brain. When Mum was at high school in that same Connecticut town, she remembers 'A breeze that snaps the flag on the flagpole and shimmers trees in the empty forecourt'. What a lonely, windblown sound.

'Lonely' is different from 'alone'. When I am alone is when I hear some of my most comforting sounds. The trucks changing gears on the nearby highway, a faraway, curling rumble that tells me the world is moving as it should. The peculiar Australian chorus of currawongs, crows and magpies – ringing, cawing, warbling – that means I never forget how far away from the rest of the world Australia is.

There's that silence, too – the absence of sound that creates memories just as keenly. The dead phone waiting for a doctor to ring. The closed door with an apology unmoved behind it. Five thousand souls on the dock by Buzz's ship:

> *One night we were showing movies on the deck [of the USS Jenkins]. The side of the dry-dock wasn't more than twenty feet from the side of the ship. We started showing when there was still a bit of light, and there had been no-one around. It got dark while we were watching the movie. In the middle, changing the reels, the lights were turned on. There were at least five thousand locals standing on the dock. They had been watching the film too. There*

were women, with babies in arms and they had not made one sound as they walked up and stood. Not one sound.

I know I won't forget my echoic memories, because my forebears didn't forget theirs either. They have catalogued their small sounds, their non-sounds, and their soundtracks of background nothingness. These interludes that worm into our consciousness and help us remember. Grama listened hard, in East Africa:

Njiroge was the old Kikuyu [garden hand] who came with the house. Years before he had worked with the owner in landscaping the property and now he regarded that particular acre of Africa as his domain. Every morning as I was having my second cup of coffee the sound of his sweeping would drift in through the open window. Each day he cut a new broom, a besom of scented herbs that smelled as well as sounded soothing as he brushed the rough stone steps.

Lesson #163: Listen. Sit still, and really listen.

Now you're listening, it's time to play. Your father loves music. He loves it with an obsession that I thought I shared, until I met him. But mine is a mere crush compared with Tom's undying love affair. He will fall in love with a musician, and dive into their back catalogue like a suitor possessed. So much so that each artist, album or song of that period has become a musical cornerstone of our lives together. In the early days, there were sweaty gigs in rooms filled with smoke and limbs, dotted across London. Later, albums circuited through our home as we fed you, cleaned with you, danced with you. While I mightn't be able to hold a tune, I know I've definitely been a part of your musical education so far. You have a back catalogue knowledge better than many thrice your age. You too, agree that the B-Side of *Abbey Road* is better.

Lesson #164: Anyone who prefers the A-Side of **Abbey Road** *is wrong.*

I've seen less live music than my husband and my mother – both of whom understand that world of performance much better than I do. Yet there are a few gigs that sit glowing in my heart, that I'll never let go.

There were Tom and I at the Brixton Academy to see The Killers play their last gig before they became stadium famous. Brandon Flowers strutted with the bravado that only a frontman with that name, and that eyeliner, can possess. Yet I was so intoxicated by Tom that I barely noticed.

Favourite song: 'Mr Brightside'.

(If you had to ask me what 'our' song was, Tom and I would tell you 'Mr Brightside'. Which is odd because it's a track about infidelity, jealousy and loss. But more about that later.)

In 2005, I'd been living with Tom long enough to embed Paul Kelly into the correct locations in his body (heart, head, stomach). I was breathless to hear he was playing a tiny gig at the Spitz by Spitalfields Market. Once there, I drank too much white wine, giddy at my proximity to this Australian legend. I'm afraid I stood too close to the little stage, singing every lyric while (probably) staring directly at his face. Smooth, Ella.

Lesson #165: Your mother was never cool.

If Paul noticed the mooning fan, he didn't show it – instead he scowled at the drunk Poms talking loudly at the bar, oblivious to the living legend rolling out his classics in their vicinity.

Like most Melburnians, I've had a few close encounters with Paul Kelly. I've never spoken to him, which – let's be honest – is probably for the best.

One summer's eve in the mid-1990s, Mum and I were hovering in the lamplit quadrangle of my brother's school. It was a fundraising event and Mum had asked me to come along as her date, to avoid another turn as a single mother in a sea of smug-marrieds. Across the crowd we spied the unmistakable head of Mr Kelly himself. Mum sent your Uncle Jim, who was a mere primary school boy, over to get his autograph. She was too shy and I was too mortified and Jim was neither. When my brother returned with a slip of paper, the pen-scrawl read:

Shame on you, making a boy do a woman's work. Paul Kelly.

I think we both privately fell in love with Paul Kelly then. Although for me, I didn't realise I had until a good ten years later.

Favourite song: Is it 'Melting', or 'If I Could Start Today Again'? Maybe 'Petrichor', but surely 'Careless'? … Don't ask me to pick one.

In 2016 Tom and I flew to Sydney to see Crowded House at the Sydney Opera House. I had recorded their 1996 performance at the same location on cassette. Twenty years later and here we were – standing up close, before the stage I'd listened to on repeat for twenty years. Your parents got joyfully drunk and ended up eating fried squid afterwards in Chinatown after midnight, electrified by the proximity we'd experienced to musical greatness.

Favourite song: 'Italian Plastic'. It's the harmonies.

If you want to make a movie night of it, you can pull up the broadcast of that 2016 performance. Tom and I sang every Crowded House lyric, danced with our fingers reaching up to the stars and the bats circling the lights, and were captured doing it all on the live coverage. There we are – four rows back and towards the Botanic Gardens.

You'll also want to get a hold of the original Woodstock festival film. No, we weren't there (this family is good at time travelling, but not *that* good). Your grandmother Kate was though. Mum was sixteen and had driven with her best friend to the dairy farm to check out the music festival they'd heard about. They didn't tell Kate's parents, Buzz and Virginia, where they were going – thinking they'd be back within twenty-four hours.

It was a heaving, muddy mess of endless people who were not all peace, love and understanding. Kate and her best friend couldn't get out for four days:

I just want to go home.

Rotten mud that smells. Filthy, trampled grass and the waft of smoke. I'm so, so hungry.

'Hey cherry pie, you got any cigarettes?' He's taller than his friends and wears a blanket over his head. He's smiling and his face is pitted. He looks gnarly like the Wicked Witch – with sideburns.

'We don't smoke.' I try to sound older than sixteen. I also try hard not to sound scared. I've been doing this since Friday and mostly these psychos give up and go away. Go on, go away and pester someone else – there's a good hippie.

His friend, Blond Bandana Boy is suddenly right up close, and yells, 'GIVE HIM YOUR CIGARETTES YOU DUMB BITCH.' He sways gently forward into my face, then back.

… I just want to go home.

Tom and I have many more live music joys.

Bon Iver in a basement below Bourke Street, a room so small we could hear his sigh when the mic cut out. Paul McCartney making a stadium *feel* that small, for the brief spell when he played 'Blackbird'. Elbow's soaring rendition of 'One Day Like This' at The Palace Theatre also on Bourke Street, Melbourne, making me cry under the disco ball lights.

Falling in love with Bruce Springsteen in a devotional performance at Hanging Rock, when I understood quickly and intensely why Tom would be seeing him three times in the same tour.

Lesson #166: Live music feeds the soul.

One of the best things about a live gig is feeling the bass in your chest while you sing louder than you've ever done before. The very best thing is: no-one else can hear you sing.

I do not sing well. At primary school there was the brutally named Special Choir, which only accepted members who had passed an audition. That was, until you were in Grade Six, when those who had failed the audition (me) could enter without trial (me again). I was so excited to join the group of choristers that when the music teacher took me aside after the first rehearsal and asked me to, 'Just … mouth the words', I didn't mind.

When Virginia wrote about her father, Jim, it seems that my (lack of) talent may have someone else to blame:

> *The separate dining room had double glass doors leading to the living room where there was a baby grand piano which Daddy played with great verve and little talent. He was completely tone deaf and could happily play an entire piece with his hands one key to the right or left of the correct position. He would sing as he played songs from his university days, wartime and current hits. It [all] sounded fine to him.*

You, on the other hand, can hold a tune. You take after your father. Both of you: an ear for a lyric, harmony and key that you may have only heard once before. Did you know your dad was in a band? But he's never sung for us, not properly. Make him sing for you; maybe he'll do it if you ask him nicely.

Music is part of our home and our family and us. Your father and I both grew up with sound from records, cassettes and CDs, both ours and our parents'. They were discovering their music in the 1960s and listened as history came through the radio. At sixteen, Kate received that kiss from Jim Morrison, as well as a drumstick from Sly and the Family Stone. And, of course, our grandparents listened to Sinatra and Vera Lynn.

Buzz and Virginia were married in 1951, and slow-danced for forty-four years:

The wedding was low-key and beautiful. One of Mother's friends played 'our' song on the piano, 'I Know Where I'm Going', then the wedding march.

*

Buzz died at Shenzi in Point Lonsdale in 1995, aged seventy. Buzz and Virginia had three children, five grandchildren, and – at the time of writing – six great-grandchildren. He is buried high on the hill in Point Lonsdale cemetery. When we visit we look out to the Rip and the Bay. Buzz's name is spoken out loud, often, and with love.

We were in love until the day he died.
I'm still in love with him.

*

The moment light truly cracked through the clouds for me, as a mother, occurred because of a song. This time, it was around the 5 pm slump, when the length of a day home alone with a baby had built up to almost too much. When caffeine, sugar and the wonder of you could no longer stem the tide of my loneliness.

We were in our little cottage in Windsor, where the kitchen was bigger than our London flat, but still small enough to also be the dining and living room. I strapped you into the baby bouncer, and I lifted you up, bouncer and all, to set you in the middle of the small kitchen table. You were almost at eye level with me, and those enormous blue ones of yours widened at the shift in your angle. I put on music. Loud, adult music and I sang loudly enough to stop us both crying. I was beginning to understand there was no rule book for motherhood and if I chose to, I could write some rules of my own. This was a very important realisation. As I sang, chopped vegetables and danced, you started to laugh. Your legs straightened and bent to bounce, and your arms flapped and you *laughed*. I started to laugh too, hysterically, then genuinely. Then wholeheartedly. I played the 'End of the Line' four times and that was the moment when I realised everything was going to be fine.

Lesson #167: Sing.

Music is emotion, injected straight into your veins. And not just the memories of emotion, with notes dredging up old times. No, the initial listen can be as enchanting as the hundredth. The precise magic of hearing a song for the very first time and being lifted – lifted – LIFTED – high up. It's like nothing else.

It's like falling in love at first sight and singing their name in your sleep. It's being obsessed with the speckle of melody that has hit you hard and you want to eat it up and swallow it down.

It is me, swooping down Punt Road filled-fresh with the news of a clear MRI ('No cancer', my oncologist wrote). Waving my hands to a honey-thick voice reverberating around my car. I flew past the winterbare trees of Gosch's Paddock, and over the gurgling brown Yarra. I flew all the way home to you on that song that told me there was heaven in me, now, in that very moment.

As we prepare to die, the last sense to fade is sound. If we cannot speak, if we cannot see, even if we cannot feel the touch at our fingertips – we can hear.

Lean in, whisper to me, my love. Sound me a story. Sing me a song.

Lesson #168: No matter where I am, I will always be listening.

Letter Twenty-five

Be ready for what love can do

The first time I saw your father, I was sitting in the courtyard of that converted toffee factory. That office that rambled over three floors, higgledy-piggledy back stairs, secret rooms and of course, that enormous kitchen in the basement. And that is where I was gazing back into when He walked across the floor. I'm sure it's Vaseline on my psychic lens, but I'm still certain that even where I sat, outside looking in, I noticed his eyes.

His eyes.

Oh, his blue, blue eyes.

I am going to embarrass you in this letter, because I am going to talk to you about loving your father. And that will include some bits about how absolutely magnetic I found him. How tempting, how addictive and how – eventually – impossible-to-ignore …

You might get squeamish, I don't know. I don't know what it is like to have a father and mother love one another, and talk about magnetism, and temptation. What I *do* know, is that when I read the heart-thuddingly raw love letters between Jim and Kay, I feel no embarrassment. Enough time has passed for the inter-generational squeamishness to have disappeared from letters such as this:

> *So many, many times, when I've shivered in a shell-hole, with my knees in six inches of water, and Fritzie sending young boxcars over my head every ten seconds, I've wondered if I ever would see your dear face again – and you've seemed nearer to me in those moments when you were farthest away.*
>
> *I've seen your face – always with the lashes of your eyes half lowered, as if half ashamed to show their glorious message. It was so you looked at me in the lights of a California sunset on the Point at Alum Rock in April, 1917 – remember – when you turned from me toward the valley and breathed – 'Glory' in a way I shan't forget.*

Breathing a single word in a way a man can't forget means one thing: a fire that burned bright and hot enough that their love endured until the day Kay died.

*

Kay passed away peacefully at her home in 2001, aged 105. She and Jim left behind three children, fourteen grandchildren, and many great and great-greats. Kay's name is spoken aloud often, and with love.

*

Maybe we agree, you and I, that if you squint your eyes and angle your head just so, you can read this letter as a love story. And not the people who you see with eyes un-squinted: people who are wrinkled and muddled in dressing gowns, making school lunches. If it's too hard to avoid the yuck-factor, then you can skip over this letter until you yourself are wrinkled and muddled. I'm sure you'll look to our love story with much kinder eyes, then.

*

The next time I was aware of Tom after the blue-eyed strut across the cafe floor was one evening, late at work. He was sitting at a desk and handing over a small project to me before he took a week off. Did I mention he was my boss? I mean, he wasn't – but he was, technically, a more senior version of the role I had interviewed over and over for. Even then I had the sense that your father was a terrible Account Man. He'll cheerfully admit it now. Honestly, I think he'd cheerfully admit it then. At that agency Tom spent a lot of time playing darts with the handyman, smoking cigarettes by the dozen and flirting with most of the office. Your father was a terrible flirt.

Lesson #169: There is absolutely nothing wrong with being a flirt.

Back to the evening in the office. Tom was off to some exotic location and I had crouched down next to him to look at his laptop. Our knees touched briefly and my stomach flipped and that's when I knew I was in trouble. At the time, I was living with another man – the one I had moved my life 16,000 kilometres for. This was shitty timing and an unplanned-for feeling. Also, due to my father's own history, I had an aversion to any kind of infidelity. I still do.

So, Tom and I circled around one another, flirting in a harmless way until it didn't feel harmless at all and I realised I was pushing the definition of infidelity closer and closer to the ledge I swore I'd never leap from.

> *Infidelity | noun*
> *Sitting on a sofa in a small flat in Camden with your Nokia 6210, typing out text messages you're pretty sure your boyfriend wouldn't want to read.*

Lesson #170: Don't beat yourself up about being a shit in your twenties.

I am not proud of how I behaved when Tom and I first met. I was young and dumb and I was falling in love with one man while still loving another. There were months of messiness. I had left the Top Floor Flat and the boy in Camden, and decided I would be single. I then spent an entire spring and some of summer mentally careering between two men. I was telling myself that because I wasn't sleeping with both of them (and I wasn't), this made it all okay (it didn't).

Lesson #171: Regardless of how old you aren't, try not to be too much of a shit.

I won't lie to you. Those new, heady days were fun. Even once I'd left my relationship, my flat, my entire reason for being in London, Tom and I were still colleagues. I made a – frankly – pathetic attempt to stay away from him and his blue, blue eyes. This was made much more difficult by the fact that we were sitting opposite each other in the office. I gave up, we started dating, but decided it would be best to keep our courtship to ourselves. Which meant we spent three months kissing in crooked alleys and dark bars and thinking no-one at work knew what we were doing.

(Spoiler 1: everyone knew what we were doing.)

(Spoiler 2: no-one cared.)

Beyond the snogging and the endless text messages and the knowledge that there was someone in the office who had seen me naked (disturbing, then novel, then strangely ordinary), there was something else occurring between Tom and me.

The feeling of falling for your father was also a feeling of falling for myself. I had never been with anyone who was so … dazzled by me. He listened to my words, hung on my sound, and hungered for me. We stayed up until dawn. We rolled in fresh sheets. We pulled stories and truths from each other like knotted Christmas lights. We started to undo them, together.

Lesson #172: The love of a good person can make you realise you are a good person.

After break-ups and back-togethers, Tom and I really, actually, did break up. Even as I watched his face sink, I couldn't stop the words that were coming out of my mouth. I left him at a bus stop on Regent Street, his eyes turned low. I thought I had done something so terrible in leaving one man for another that I decided I didn't deserve to be with either of them. This was both illogical and stupid.

Lesson #173: Self-flagellation does not serve anyone well.

I missed everything about Tom, but I still thought it was the Right Thing To Do. He went to a music festival and moped on everyone's shoulder. I lay in my basement room and wondered if it was normal to feel like my heart had turned to cinders. We had deleted each other from our phones (this was tantamount to dying in the years before social media). And then – one night – we came back together.

I had written Tom's number on a small piece of paper and hidden ('hidden') it from myself in my desk. One night, after the cinders piled too high, I started scrabbling in drawers looking for a white flag of notepaper. I found it, I waved it and Tom came. He tells me he was sitting in his newly purchased flat and watched my number flash and flash and flash on the phone screen. He wondered if he should pick it up. If this mad Australian girl was worth all the mess.

'I …' I was crying, 'I think I've made a mistake.'

Your father made a dramatic late-night taxi run to rescue me, soggy with tears, slumped on the black and white-tiled forecourt in Marylebone. Finally, Tom and I clicked into the same gear at the same time. That night was a new beginning, when our love suddenly felt … permanent. I like to mark August 31, 2004, as our anniversary. Your father says one's wedding anniversary should rescind all previous commemorations.

Lesson #174: Your mother is always right.

From that August day we were In Love and it was a feeling of being simultaneously deeply comforted and thrillingly excited. There was a fantastic proper pub around the corner from Tom's Belsize Square flat, with sticky carpet, low embroidered stools and golden lighting. Sean Bean drank there a lot. Years later, when I saw him appear on my screen in *Game of Thrones*, I was transported back to pints of Stella and the curious citrus smell in the Belsize Tavern toilets. We spent a lot of our early relationship in that pub, talking, feeling each other's futures out. It was in there that I told Tom that I was a true-blue, dinky-di Aussie and I would most certainly be going back to Australia one day.

He, in his own words, 'chose to ignore that bit'.

*

There have been three seminal moments in your parents' relationship. None of these has included marriage or (sorry) you. But they have led to these things, built them up, and held them there.

Lesson #175: Your parents are people, too.

The first was a long weekend in Rome. We sat on the bed in a hotel room under the Aventine Hill, the sun going down through the trees outside. The branches were heavy with oranges and the dusk made them glow an even deeper amber.

This was years after moving in together, and we had been dancing around the fact that I wanted to return to Australia, and that Tom had said he wanted to come with me. And that only one of those things was true. It was a conversation we had avoided and avoided and now, as I picked at the label on my bottle of Moretti, I realised with a gut-churn that this was the Conversation. Where it was going to end. Or not.

That was the conversation that brought us to Australia.

I recall thinking that even as we told each other that we loved one another; that we very much wanted to get married and have babies and live happily ever after … that it mightn't work out. That I might wing my way back to the homeland and Tom would … not. And with a lump in my throat as we headed off for a late Roman supper, exhausted from Crying and Deciding, a very small voice said,

'Go home. Alone. If he doesn't follow, it wasn't meant to be.'

Back in our tree-cast flat in Belsize I sat on an Ikea stool and booked my one-way ticket back to Australia.

'There,' I said, as I closed the lid of the laptop.

He would have been watching TV. Smartphones didn't exist then.

'Hmm?' Distracted.

I swivelled on the stool. Slightly too-low, knees bent. Looked at those blue eyes.

'I've booked it. I've done it.'

Tom looked wounded and surprised, and that's your dad, my love. He is eternally optimistic and can be distracted by that optimism. And I knew that, even at twenty-five, it would be me who had to book that plane ticket, and hope that he would eventually do the same.

That afternoon in Rome wasn't significant because it was the moment we decided to be together, but because it was the conversation that led to me leaving. It was the moment we realised work would need to be put in, and that we – together – were worth it. If I'd stayed in London, my resentment would have grown along with my sadness. If I'd provided Tom an ultimatum to fly home with me, then and there, then his journey would have begun with emotional coercion. We both had to leave London on our own terms, which we did – just, five months apart.

Lesson #176: Together does not always mean 'at the same time'.

*

The second moment was that evening of my thirtieth birthday, overnight in that almost locked-up bed and breakfast in Queenscliff. Over dinner we had eaten duck tongues (small, salty, delicious) and talked about leaving IVF behind and moving to Italy. Bubbles of happiness blew big in my chest. It had been a long time since we were so excited about the future. That was the night we both agreed that we would be living a life without the child we wanted, and that we were going to be okay.

I don't subscribe for one second to the idea that 'giving up trying means you'll get pregnant' or anything else that suggests medical success (pregnancy, cancer cures) can be controlled by the mind. The reason for this is it's just so cruel. It suggests those who can't ever have a child, or who die from cancer, just didn't want the alternative enough. This night in Queenscliff wasn't significant because it's the night you were conceived (it was – sorry), but because it's the night Tom and I agreed our love was enough. That each other, was enough.

That was the conversation that brought us to you.

Lesson #177: Be ready to fall in love with Plan B.

The third was in the back yard in our house when Tom was ill. Iller than either of us had realised and I was having the cold creep of understanding that there was no other grown-up standing in the yard to fix it. It was just us. It was just me.

Tom had severe enough anxiety that it was impacting our marriage, him, and you. That conversation on that day saw him reach up and out of his own illness, and do so because of his love for you, and for me and – most importantly – for himself. That was the day that he started to seek help and it was one of the bravest things I've ever seen anyone do. That was the conversation that brought him back to us.

Lesson #178: Accepting help can be harder than offering it. Do both.

Your parents' love affair began with such *drama*, a diamond created through the shifting tectonic plates of text messages and tears. I was addicted to Tom. And little wonder. Meeting him and getting to know him was a bigger journey than any of the kilometres from Melbourne to London. Meeting Tom was meeting a man with wit and wonder: he was clever unlike anyone else I'd loved before. We sat in bars and lay on picnic rugs and cuddled into each other on trains and we talked in ways that felt surgical. Nothing was left. Every story he told, I held to myself like an organ he'd removed from his own body. It sounds revolting, but falling in love is revolting. It is that knitted skin. It is the bloody merging of two souls until they're so enmeshed that any separation will cause pain and death.

When you were born you looked entirely like Tom and nothing like me. The evolutionary folklore goes that 'a newborn resembles its father to prevent him from abandoning the cave'. This has been disproved, but the rule could have assisted us, in the opposite direction. Because if anyone was likely to do any abandoning in those brand-new days, it was me. Although I think the anxiety and exhaustion wouldn't have been helped by you looking like your mother. And anyway, it's good, because you inherited your father's eyes.

What you now display in attributes from your father, I hope you keep. Because he has so many good ones. He devours books, film and song as if his life was made from those things. You recently started to read until 10 pm which is probably much too late for a nine-year-old. But honestly, I'm just glad I'm done with years of calling down the hall 'Go to sleep!'

Lesson #179: It's okay to stay up past your bedtime when a book is to blame.

Tom can hold a tune and a harmony, and retains a picture-perfect image of those and lyrics, and so can you. So now, in between the two of you songbirds I remain a honking, tuneless goose.

Tom is handsome. He is funny. He draws better than I. He is clever in a casual, 'I just threw this together' sort of way, which is as irritating as it is impressive.

But the most astounding thing about your father is how kind he is. He is a good man. The older we all get the more I realise just how important and valuable these qualities are.

Like any long relationship, the fury and flame has died down. Now, seventeen years after falling into each other for the last, first time, Tom and I – glow.

Sigh. I'm sorry – I can't talk about a long-term relationship without falling into clichés.

And what clichés we had. We had grand gestures, twenty-page love letters and afternoons spent with slow sex and naps and drinking beer before sunset. We had Paris, and Rome and an engagement in the treetops overlooking the biggest horizon I'd ever seen. We had grief and fear and simmering resentments. We had long, long months of nothing at all. We had all those things.

But the grandest of grand gestures, the most romantic and passionate and extraordinary thing is something you, yourself, see every day. Your father left his life. His family. His friends. His world. He left it all behind and every day he is without them is a day staked in the ground that declares a greater love than I could have ever hoped for.

I'm sharing all this because this is a love letter to your father, but it is also for you.

I do not know what it feels like to have parents who love each other.

I don't want you to feel doubt if ever you're in the same position.

I hope one day you can have a love like ours.

Lesson #180: Fall in love with someone you can say that about.

You don't grow up a child of a many-divorced couple with stars in your eyes about marriage and love. I always wonder if this might be 'our last decade' as a married couple, not because anything is wrong, but because I know wrong can always appear around the corner.

Tom is the opposite. His parents were married long and deeply, until his dear, beloved father died. And that is his expectation for us, that we will remain enmeshed until death splits us in two. The longer we remain together, the more history we pack into our combined souls, the more I think he might be right. On the night we split up for the last time, back in 2004, Tom wrote to me:

> *We both know how we feel about one another. I have to be confident that you won't forget that … And you have to believe me when I say I'm not going anywhere. And we both have to believe that this story will have a happy ending, whatever that ends up meaning.*

Lesson #181: Your father is always right.

Letter Twenty-six

Terrible things will occur

We are getting close to the end. And now is time for me to write you one of my last letters.

As I have been doing throughout, I place the noise-cancelling headphones over my ears. Before I turn on the music – or the white noise, or whatever it is I'm listening to – the outside world is blanked out and I can hear myself breathing.

In. Out. In. Out.

And I am reminded of scuba diving. Spacewalking. Dying. I don't know for sure, but in every movie I've seen that has included those activities, this is exactly what it's sounded like.

In. Out. In. Out.

I am down in the deepest watery trench for you. I am floating, untethered, in the white-light of space for you. I am dying for you.

Flick my oxygen switch, daughter of mine – we're going in.

I have shown you craters and wounds. Buildings have tumbled, mothers have fallen, men have been blown up.

This is a letter about standing tall again, covered in the dust and the pieces.

When Jim was injured in Belgium, the shrapnel hit his right arm, shoulder and chest. It was a critical wound and a number of horses and men around him were killed:

> *Shortly afterward the entire northern end of Belgium rose and stood on end. I recollect rising in the air, out of the saddle, and then next thing I remember was someone poking my ribs and saying, in an uncouth voice: 'Hell! He can still grunt when you kick 'im. He must be alive.'*

With his beloved mare, Betty, nowhere to be seen, Jim and his orderly (who was also wounded in the same blast) began to pick their way back to their own lines, and then eventually to a first-aid station. In the field, this station was typically a little farmhouse with planks instead of beds, operated by half a dozen 'corpsmen', or medicos:

> *They put me up on the planks, and gave me an injection or two of anti-tetanus, and fixed me up and told me to get down. [As] my orderly got up … an Austrian .88 shell hit this house [and] it blew the roof off. Now, whenever a shell or an earthquake hits a house or a room that is plaster, you can't see for about twenty minutes. Everything comes down in dust and pieces.*
>
> *When it cleared away, I looked around, and the medical corpsmen had all disappeared. We never did see one of them again. I found out later that they were new men who had never been under fire before, so they just took off.*
>
> *I finished tying up the orderly, which wasn't much trouble. His wound was slight; he'd just had the calf of one leg sort of sheared.*

When bad things happen to you, there are three types of people: those who run away, those who freeze, and those who bend down and tie up your wound. A trick to joining the last group can be swapping fear for curiosity. It doesn't always work, but even the smallest attempt can be success in itself. Do you remember when Jim was eleven and an earthquake came to knock the fronts from the houses?

> *[It] shook that house of ours, the new house, off its foundations. It didn't hurt the water mains; we had water, if we capped the leaky taps, which … my father was able to do right away. And [so] we cooked breakfast on our bonfire in the yard. …*

My darling, I can tell you now that if all the fronts fell off all the houses and we were having breakfast on a bonfire in our yard, I would not be letting you wander uptown to pick over piles of brick and doll's house homes. But if I did, I would hope that you would be as interested – and therefore, as protected – as your great-great-grandfather was. Being Interested is the best tool against fear that I can give to you. Your great-great-grandfather clearly knew this, even at eleven years old.

Lesson #182: If you're interested, you're less likely to be scared.

When I was diagnosed with cancer, I decided to document everything I could, and share it to both strangers and friends on the internet. (This is probably the most 2020s statement you'll read in any of these letters: I apologise.) But it really helped, my girl. Sharing the interesting parts of what was happening to me was a wonderful shield against the horrible things my days included.

I began as I meant to go on: I announced my illness on Instagram. I built a slide show in pastels and emojis that finished with a helpful Q&A instructing people how *I* wanted *them* to react to my news.

> *If you see me in the school playground please, put away the Pity Eyes. I don't need them, thanks. However, both humour and nakey Jude Law pics gratefully received.*

It worked. That weekend, my phone pinged with Nudey Judey night and day. After a bleak fortnight, I smiled for forty-eight hours straight.

Lesson #183: If you're laughing, you're less likely to be scared.

I was embarrassed to be diagnosed with anal cancer. ANAL. It's not a gentle word, no matter how you say it. Not only is the word confronting, but the treatment is brutal and the side-effects can be ferocious.

In the early days, when I had to tell people over and over what was wrong with me, I craved the relative grace of 'breast'.

I learned how to manage it for them, when they asked, 'Can I ask what cancer you had, Ella?'

Lights up, girls! Eyes bright. Eyebrows high.

'Ooh, it's a gross one – are you ready?'

Wait a beat, maybe two – are they prepared?

'Anal. I had anal cancer.'

Slap 'em with a big grin. Hit the music. Exit stage left.

By the tenth time I had the routine down pat. Now, I'm a veritable 1000-show Vegas veteran. I'd do anything to keep people from looking at me the way I looked at me when I was first diagnosed.

What's that, Jim?

> *Oh, I have always hammed everything up; sometimes it produces great benefits. And, if it doesn't, they just laugh at you, and that doesn't hurt anything.*

When I was admitted to hospital for pain management, your father and I sat in the waiting room of the cancer ward. It was filled with the funeral services of former patients, presented like Christmas cards on a really, really sad mantelpiece. It was surreal and horrific and we were giggling by the time the nurse returned with my paperwork. The pastel shades of the quiet hospital seems nothing compared to the mud and rain of no-man's-land, but (if I'd been reading them at the time) I know Jim's words would have still managed to comfort me.

> *I've seen a whole lot of concentrated war in the last few weeks, and I can't say that I enjoyed every minute of it. There were times, lots of them, when I felt a sort of exultation – a kind of rejoicing in the fact that the thing was so hard – a desire to test how much of it I could look at, and still laugh. A lot of that old feeling that you and I know so well came to me: that joy of breasting something and coming through, and I'm ready for more of it, which, from all indications, I'll get.*

Hospital was the point when my oversharing hit a particularly hysterical stride. I was moving through waves of 11/10 pain that would last for hours, making my ears ring and my vision go white. I was also watching a lot of *Grand Designs*.

In those weeks, I was overmedicated, understimulated and more scared than I had ever been in my life. I figured that if I could get a laugh out of this, I could get a laugh out of anything.

Posting my experiences online reframed some of the really bad stuff. It was the ultimate distraction. I went through treatment seeking out the funny, the curious, the new – thinking about how to share it in a fifteen-second grab. I didn't have time to be nervous when I was filming a time-lapse of my first radiation treatment. I didn't weep in loss after a bustling nurse waved a pink 'vaginal dilator' in front of my husband's raised eyebrows. I couldn't vomit with fear when I was joking about Tom's 'motivational music' ahead of my first post-treatment scan.

Remember what I said about self-awareness? I want to tell you something in case, one day, you are wondering.

I knew.

I knew every piece of my pain shared on the internet was something I would be judged for. I knew it was obnoxious, and cringey and self-involved. But – and this is the best bit – I didn't care.

I still don't.

The best thing about explosions, pain and white-eyed fear is this: you don't give a shit anymore.

Lesson #184: Nothing is more powerful than a woman who no longer gives a shit.

Grama said that we were 'a family who believed they were important enough'.

I started these letters wondering if I was 'enough' to join them. But now, twenty-six letters down, I'm realising that it doesn't really matter. At least, not to anyone but you and me.

I want you to stop caring. Been kicked? Grunt back. Give no shits, bend down, tie up that wound and ride your motherfucking horse out of there, because life is short and no-one cares about you as much as you care about you.

Oh, didn't I mention? Jim's horse, Betty, survived the artillery attack as well.

> *[The orderly] and I helped each other toward the door. When we opened the door, there stood Betty, my horse, waiting for me. She was clear up to her withers in mud; she'd been out in the fields, and followed us along the road as the orderly and I came back. Then she had come up to the door, waiting. And she stayed there during this shelling. She was wounded; she had a three-cornered tear in her right rump, like a tear in canvas. But otherwise she wasn't crippled, and she could walk, and was all right.*
>
> *... Now [Betty] wears a blue ribbon in her halter, and is almost as proud of it as I am. She's entitled to one service stripe,*

one wound stripe, and a blue ribbon, and that's more than most veterans can claim.

I have four radiation tattoos, a postmenopausal body, laparoscopic scars from IVF and a removed-appendix, and enough PTSD to keep five Instagram accounts full.

These are banners, medal and ribbons I wear with pride.

Lesson #185: Honour the stripes you earn with pride.

You lucky, sad, brave girl. Your mother might be gone, but you have an entire army of noisy ancestors behind you and beside you. I trust by now you believe me when I say: we remain ready to teach you, bore you, lift you up, make you laugh and ensure you will never, ever be lost.

You see, that is what this collection has been for. For me to say goodbye, and for you to continue without me. For you to believe there is always the chance that you will feel love, and light and happiness again.

And that chance is the reason to keep going.

Lesson #186: Keep. Going.

*

Jim passed away peacefully at his Palo Alto home in 1989, aged 94. He left his Kay, their three children, fourteen grandchildren, and many great and great-greats. Jim's name is spoken aloud often, and with love.

*

As I've written to you, I've been reading the family letters and memoirs over and over, many times. I think Jim would be chuffed to hear that one of my favourite quotes is his. I can apply it to almost anything I've withstood, up until now. I hope it will help you, too:

> *I think – that if I ever get back – this affair will have done me a lot of good. Happiness, as they say, is never appreciated unless it is paid for.*

Lesson #187: Happiness is never appreciated unless it is paid for.

Letter Twenty-seven

Know this

The last goodbye. The last letter.

This is a wonderful way for me to tell you: 'I am still here.'

I did not die.

Just yet.

So far.

Now, as of this moment, I am still alive, kicking and here to share myself and my (your) family with you.

There is one lesson I have taught myself, in the writing of my letters and the reading of others:

Lesson #188: Tell your stories.

Share your words before it is too late. Say everything over and over so there is no doubt. Write them down and call them out into the sky. And so, to follow my own instruction, here are some final words, some for now, most for when the day comes that I am gone.

Know how fiercely I love you. How dazzled and amazed I am by you. How completely I forgive you, for what I do not know – but for everything you wonder about from today until your own dying moment: I absolve you.

Know how burstingly proud I am of you, of your talents now and the ones I haven't seen yet. Know how excited I am for you and your future. Know I am excited for your father's future too. His love, which is so precious, will find its way to someone new. Be kind to them. Be kind to him. Love them, if that's what you'd like to do. Let them love you, if that's what you need.

Know how hard I fought to stay here for you. How I kicked, bit, scrambled and crawled my way for another year – day – breath – to be with you. Know you are the reason for everything, and for nothing at all. Feel the weight of my love but feel utterly freed of any requirement or legacy. I expect nothing of you, except to be kind to yourself.

Know that you are the only person who can be truly kind to yourself. Speak with the love and gentle humour I know you have, and use your words on your own self. Tell yourself the beautiful truths I know you are capable of sharing. Do not be cruel, do not be critical. Someone who loves themselves is unstopppable. It is a power only you can bestow, but I am imploring you to use it.

Know that I'm sorry. I'm sorry for any way in which I failed you. I'm sorry for something that I have not mentioned that you may find later, that I didn't even know will make you sad. I'm sorry for hurt and for insensitivity. I'm sure I was a jerk. Know that I know.

Know that my love is so strong, and so powerful, that it stretches far beyond you and through to those you love. I love your partner. I love your child. I love the clever things that you will create. Bring them into your world and I will bring them into mine. Tell them I love them, I love them for loving you.

Know that I lived a joyous, wonderful, privileged life. For most of the time, for all of the time that really mattered – I was happy. I loved and was loved. I was boring and extraordinary and pedestrian and phenomenal. In all of this, I hope very much the intent was on the right side of the balance sheet. Because I did great things. I did not-so-great things. I did so many tiny things that did not matter. But they mattered to me, because I was alive. I was *alive*!

Finally, know that I – and all those who came before – know that *we* are in your heart and your soul and your very being, whether you like it or not.

Thank you for making me a mother. Thank you for being you, and for allowing me to say: I am not gone, ever. I am always here, for you.

I love you, my darling girl.

Mama x

Afterword

You are invited

You are invited to a party. All of you, not just you, darling daughter, but everyone. Everyone here, in this space, reading these words. Take my hand; let's go. We've been waiting.

You've received an invitation. It has arrived on heavy stock. You're not sure how your address is known: nobody posts mail anymore. Your name is written with a deep-blue ink. The envelope smells very faintly of lemons.

The guests have been told to arrive at an innocuous address in a city you've always wanted to visit. The sun is only half an hour from setting, which is excellent, because it has been very hot today and you don't want to sweat your hair wet again. As you arrive, all you can see is a long, long wall lit dimly with lanterns swinging slightly in the evening breeze. Somewhere, you can hear a sprinkler. A dog barks. You smell sausages. Strange place to have a party, an unpaved road where the houses are too large to be seen from the footpath.

As you're about to wave the car back to you, you realise there *is* a door here. It's bedded into the wall and looks older than any you've walked through in a while. The timber is dark and heavy and there's a brass knocker that is also dark and –

oh? – no chance to feel if it's heavy as well – it's opening. You're going in.

After a hushed exchange in which you give your name to the woman who doesn't seem to need a clipboard, you're waved off vaguely in the direction you're to walk. It feels much later in the day, on the other side of the wall. The trees are tall enough to block out any of the last afternoon light. There's a path picked out from the moss: rounded stones lit by low lights, curving its way through a … your eyes widen. This can't be. Your car had barely left the town's limits but you seem to have found yourself in a lush, thick wood. Before your eyes can adjust any more, the door opens again and behind you, more guests are welcomed. You walk on into the trees.

The path winds and winds. Long enough that you stop hearing the road and can only smell the garden coming to life in the sink of the sun. Thinking back, you couldn't have walked for as long as you remember. It can't be, given this is just a garden. But in the middle of the trek, with the low murmur of the couple behind you – it feels as if you've come very far from where you started.

Then, faintly: music. Yes, you can hear it now, it's silky and rhythmic and metallic and soft at the same time. You begin to hear laughter, see lights. Hundreds of lights, glowing – bobbing – swinging. And here you are. A garden in name only, when really it feels like a golden glow of sparkle in the midst of a deep green sigh.

There's a home in the clearing you're all standing in. Although it's less house and more chateau. It is covered in a cloud of climbing roses, a lurid flush of bougainvillea and the heavy scent of jasmine. Along the base of the wall, where the bluestone meets the grass, lilac, heliotrope, gardenia and daphne mingle. You catch a shred of frangipani on the air, too. You seem to be standing in the micro-est of microclimates, where all these plants are coexisting happily.

You look left, right. It's not just the flora. The guests who surround you, and those emerging from the woods like you did, are all oddly ageless. You can't quite put your finger on it, everyone is so familiar. Everyone is so pleased to be there – it's almost as if they've never met, but have always known each other.

I'm here. Of course. I am wearing sequins and incredible shoes that are actually *extremely comfortable*, and I'm waving at you from across the garden while pointing and miming enthusiastically at the food. You don't quite understand what I'm saying, but that's okay. My hair is big and fabulous. I'm beaming.

You see a glimpse of purple through the crowd. Yes, there is Kay. Her cropped brown hair and eyes with lashes-dipped, wearing the crepe gown with spaghetti straps, skintight and flared from thigh to ankle. You suspect she's not wearing any underwear, but given she is your great-great-grandmother it's not something you dwell on for too long.

She is standing next to Jim. Of course. He's in white tails. You know it's him because there's a circle of guests tightly gathered into his story and they're hanging on every word that sparks from his smile. He is holding one of his mountain drinks and you have a feeling there may be an army pistol in his jacket pocket, for a midnight firing – as is his wont.

Kay's hand is resting gently on his arm as if to say, 'Oh, Jim.'

You hear a laugh that is carried across the crowd. There she is. The 'Professor Emeritus'. Jet-black hair coiffed in waves and a megawatt smile. Virginia is wearing that ivory brocade ball gown – there's no bottle of wine ruining the line of her dress, though – she has a glass of something gilded and fizzing in her hand instead. It's been poured by Madame Delampre, Jim's friend with the twinkling eyes. She can't speak English, but she has an abundance of drink and goodwill, both of which are flowing freely.

The sun has sunk now and you can see fireflies emerging from the trees. Although oddly, there are only two: one pink, one green. Legs, arms, iridescent wings that you feel ever-so-briefly as they shoot past your ear. You strain to hear what they are calling over the music – but it only sounds like bells. Tiny, fairylike bells.

From one of the chateau's doors comes a steady stream of waitstaff in black, a murmuration of high collars and silver trays. They are serving Kay's Bovril crisps, she has always prided herself on those – the best way to start a party off. Virginia's hors d'oeuvres have made the menu too. Stuffed olives wrapped in bacon and browned under the griller. There are smoked oysters on little toast rounds (this time, thankfully, the oven has been turned on at the correct time). Kate has contributed to the menu too. Bowls of chargrilled eggplant dip from the South Melbourne Market accompanied by toasted pita bread. I've added some items to the menu, as well – but they'll be coming later. Keep an eye out for the smoked salmon, lemon zest and horseradish blinis.

You hear a gentle snuffle and notice Betty the horse. She's delicately nibbling on the rose bushes while a pair of women exclaim over her beautiful lashes – which she is batting. Her blue ribbon is resplendent against her shining coat. Someone has plaited her mane, just so. You have a feeling she and Jim will be putting on a show before the sun is up.

The garden really is quite full now. Here's Buzz. His bald head makes him easier to pick out from all the others. He has two of his Mallet martinis, and he's passing one to your father. Tom is taking a sip and you can see his pupils enlarge with the shock of the belt of gin that's just hit the back of his throat. Buzz is leaning in, explaining something to him, and Tom's now looking mildly alarmed. You suspect he's on the receiving end of some home-brand renovation advice. Best check in on that later.

Is it that musician? It looks terribly like … It must be, because there *I* am, standing too close to the shallow stage by the side of the house, singing every lyric. Yes – it is him. And now Jim has wandered over. He is leaning one arm on a piano and singing along, a tad out of tune, but neither performer seems to mind.

The group is now moving as one and the music has lifted to another volume. It is thumping and people have begun to dance. But you are still and quiet alongside the raucous crowd. Even with the music and the movement, this feels like an especially Important Moment.

The first star has come out, a snap-frozen firework. You find yourself gazing upon it, then as your eyes lower from the sky they catch Kay's – she smiles in recognition.

Suddenly, a glimmer of gold, and it's Kate. Her blonde hair is swinging to the music and her shoes are so high you can spy her easily through the crowd. She's wearing her wedding dress and is hand-in-hand with Ross – who you notice is sporting a very fetching kilt. Boy, can those two move. They dance with the lightness of a couple who have earned it.

Buzz and Virginia drift pass, moving across the grass so smoothly that you wonder if their feet are really touching the ground.

Before you can join them your eye catches a flash of red.

There, in the furthest corner of the clearing, where the lights do not reach as brightly, you see a tent. It is Madame Mystery, with her big rings in her ears and many clinking bangles. She beckons to you with crooked hands and when you stoop your head to enter the dimness of the tent, your nose catches sawdust and canvas.

She motions for you to sit across the table from her, to gaze into the crystal ball and see what there is to see.

You decide, with a small shake of your head, to decline – and move back to the sound of the dancing and the chorus. Her dark eyes lock onto yours. She smiles.

'If you go home, you won't know what your future has in store.'

This gives you the briefest of pauses. But you don't stop. After half a breath you continue your exit. You don't need to know what your future has in store. You are armed with what your past has given you. That is enough. That is enough to keep going.

You rejoin the party. It is time to dance. The band is playing 'When I Grow too Old to Dream', and Jim and Kay are dancing: tight-framed and fluid all at the same time. Everyone is moving. There's a violin, and a saxophone. And I am there, singing and grinning with your father, forcing him to dance with me. My curly-haired husband – the one with the blue, blue eyes who made sure my story had one of the happiest of endings.

A shriek, a gale of laughter, the music pauses and then picks up again. It is moving like a wave now, in and out, the tide carrying you to the centre where children push past like kelp at your ankles. They are playing tag through legs of guests and tables, squealing with the glee of little people who know they will be staying up well past their bedtime.

You glimpse little seven-year-old Madeleina, hair ruffled as she races by. You realise with a tight suddenness that these are children who may have been lost, or had never been at all. But they are also little ones who are yet to come.

Oh, gosh. Your head is spinning – is it the champagne?

And suddenly I am there, a touch at your elbow. I told you, didn't I? No matter where I am, I will always be listening. I can see you need some air. Some altitude from the oppressive wonder that is this party of memories, lost-loves and dreams-come-true. A party that continues until the dawn, when suddenly everyone is calling everyone else's name:

'Goodnight Jim. Goodnight Kay.'

'It was the best party ever.'

'Goodnight Buzz, goodnight Male and Gladys and Birge and Lucille.'

Say them with me now: call out their names; sound out their syllables.

And you. You, holding this book of somebody else's family, who can you see? Who can you see moving through the crowd of loved ones? A shimmer of hair you remember the smell of, a wink of an eye that makes you smile, the distinctive turn of a wrist of someone you haven't held in oh-so-long? They're all here; they're all here for you and for us and for everyone for as long as they need to be. Say their names; call them out loud across the music and the dancing and the joy. Invite them to hold and remember and love you. Because they do, you know – the ones who have gone? They love you so very much.

Call out to them, through the fireflies and the moss and the rich deep green.

'Goodnight! Goodnight! We will see you again!'

And you will. Whenever you need to, you will see those who have gone, those who have come before.

Just listen to their words, carry their stories, and speak their name.

Some notes on the text

The stories in this book reflect the author's recollection of events: mine and my family's. Some (but not many) names, locations, and identifying characteristics have been changed to protect the privacy of those depicted. Dialogue has been re-created from memory.

With the permission of his wife Virginia, the decision has been made to refer to my grandfather Jim DeFriest as 'Buzz' throughout the book, although he wasn't given this nickname until the 1980s. This is for the sake of clarity, given the other Jims in the story.

List of sources

Kate Curtis, *Time Travel*, published by the author, Melbourne, Australia, 2020.

Kate Curtis, *Food Stories*, published by the author, Melbourne, Australia, 2012.

James Ellis (McDaniel) DeFriest, 'An Oral History', Point Lonsdale, 1995.

Virginia DeFriest, *No Pagodas*, Seaview Press, South Australia, 2002.

James A. Quinby, Letters to Miss Katherine Gilbert from Lt James A. Quinby, in France, Belgium and England. 24 June 1918 to 17 March 1919.

James A. Quinby, 'The Early Life of James A. Quinby as told to Will McInnis and Diana Quinby', Palo Alto, California, 1984.

Katherine Quinby, 'Family Record', Palo Alto, California, 1974.

Letter Two: contains excerpts from 2020 *Sydney Morning Herald* article: https://www.smh.com.au/lifestyle/life-and-relationships/in-1918-jim-wrote-letters-to-his-sweetheart-last-month-i-opened-them-20200423-p54mo3.html

Letter Three: the quote 'pink and purple flowers of the tinkle-tinkle tree' comes from Roald Dahl, *The Giraffe and the Pelly and Me*, Puffin Books, 2009.

Letter Six: the first time I heard the question 'What's the secret to a long marriage?' and the answer 'You don't get divorced' was by Olivia Harrison https://vimeo.com/32616278. And the quote 'Some days it's easy, some days it's hard, but when you read the words back, you can't tell which day was which' is from Neil Gaiman, https://www.masterclass.com/classes/neil-gaiman-teaches-the-art-of-storytelling

Letter Eleven: the section titled 'The empty heartbreak of longing' contains an excerpt from a 2019 'On The Spike' blog article: https://onthespike.com/2019/01/07/the-only-child/

Letter Eighteen: definition of 'coven' is from the Oxford Dictionary.

Letter Twenty: contains an excerpt from 2019 'The Grace Tales' blog article: https://thegracetales.com/ella-ward-on-why-therapy-is-not-a-dirty-word/

Letter Twenty-one: the quote 'A little party never killed nobody' is from F. Scott Fitzgerald, *The Great Gatsby*, 1925.

Letter Twenty-three: the quote that begins 'There are three deaths …' is from David M. Eagleman, *Sum: Forty Tales from the Afterlives*, Pantheon Books, 2009.

Acknowledgements

I wish I were cool enough to have a minimalist Acknowledgements page. It would contain one single, obscure sentence and you'd all wonder what it meant, while also being impressed (and relieved) at my restraint.

Sigh.

If you know me (or even if you've just read the preceding eighty-odd-thousand words) you'll know that simply will not do. So, here are all of my words:

Jim and Kay, Virginia and Buzz and my mother Kate. Thank you for allowing me to stand on your shoulders. I hope I did OK.

My publisher Catherine Milne, who reached out a hand god-knows-why and then pretended not to be alarmed when I refused to let go. Catherine, you are clever, generous and inspirational. Thank you. Thank you also to Belinda, Katie, Kristy, Dave and Lucy. You make me look good.

My agent Pippa Masson, who was extremely and unnecessarily kind when I cold-emailed you years ago. And then equally gracious when I called you back a year later yelling 'I HAVE ANOTHER BOOK THIS ONE IS BETTER PLEASE HELP ME!'

Georgie Abay, your request to publish a piece for The Grace Tales back in 2018 began this particular writing jaunt rolling – thank you for asking and then for publishing. I was still on *heavy* painkillers but it was a vibe and you went with it.

Esther Coren, you chose to politely ignore my raging girl-crush and instead provided excellent banter and a very nice cup of tea. In the weird world of social media, you kicked this all off – something I will be forever grateful for.

Jessica Dettman, a proper-proper author who has been gracious in me single-white-femaling most of your career contacts. You, my friend, are true class.

Cathrine Mahoney, your generosity and support helped me so much in the early days. I love you and your lipstick.

Simon, Alex and Lucy. You are the best and made me more happy than I'd been in such a long time. I wouldn't have been able to start this without you. To Mark and Ant, for being very handsome, charming gentlemen who didn't take it personally when I declined the Big Job Offer, and instead told you I was skipping off to write a book. You were gracious and supportive and your only condition was I referred to you as very handsome and charming in my Acknowledgements section.

All of the families and friends who make up this funny little pocket of Melbourne. You were there from when I was sick to when I was well but still not *well*-well. Thank you for the support, the childcare, the love, the text messages and the margaritas.

I wave and bow to my family members, some of whom have been included in these pages, but many who have not. My parents, my steps, my in-laws, my halves: thank you for your wisdom, your patience, your assistance and your understanding in me telling your stories.

I would also like to thank Diana McInnes and Carter Quinby, who have been enormously helpful with the American arm of the family's archives. And to my dear, special friends. Thanks for listening to me bang on and on about this for almost ever.

For those of you who are wondering if it is actually you in the book – if you liked it, yes!

If you didn't? Of course it's not.

Tom. You didn't exactly relish me parading my private parts all over Instagram, and in response I paraded more private parts all over a book. Thank you for your support. Thank you for the blue post-it note. Thank you for picking up the phone in August 2004. I love you.

And my girl. When I really thought these letters would be the only things I could leave you with, I was too scared to finish them. Thank you for giving me the best reason to fight, so now I can say – they are done.